Dmytro Kovalchuk

Invictus Equilibrium.

Immunity, Stress Resistance, and Long Life

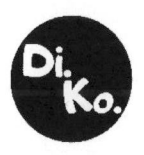

2024

Any part of this book may be copied or reproduced in any form provided the source is cited. The author believes that copyright is conditional. Any acquisition of knowledge by an individual is directly or indirectly the result of social processes, and without it (society), their acquisition is impossible in principle. A violation of copyright will be considered only the exact republication of 25% or more of the material from this book.

Contents

Foreword	4
Chapter 1. Why All This?	7
Chapter 2. Evolution Is Killing You	10
Chapter 3. Basics	14
Chapter 4. The Brain	31
Chapter 5. Sleep	50
Chapter 6. Earth	57
Chapter 7. Sun	61
Chapter 8. Water	67
Chapter 9. Air	77
Chapter 10. Body	87
Chapter 11. Nutrition	108
Chapter 12. Stimulants	145
Chapter 13. Vitamins and Minerals	159
Chapter 14. Stress	229
Afterword	239
Sources	241

Foreword

This book is not a medical manual, and I am not a doctor. Perhaps you believe that only doctors should write books about health, but I think a bit differently. Each of us knows how to prepare food, but not all of us are chefs. You don't necessarily need to be a doctor to learn to listen to your own body. Everyone should have a basic understanding of their body. This book is not about the biological knowledge of body structure - that won't be enough. This book is more about basic processes, logical connections in our body, and evolutionary adaptations that may be hard to intuitively understand at first glance but have a huge impact on our lives. This book is about things that are often very simple but can completely break your life or turn it entirely for the better.

I am an engineer. I have well-developed logic, and if you take a good look at today's classical medicine, you might conclude that it lacks a bit of it. I don't know what this is related to: politics, business, or perhaps just a one-sided view of the human body. But very often in hospitals, they treat only the consequences of diseases and completely forget about the causes. Don't get me wrong. There are plenty of extraordinarily gifted doctors who have actually saved

Invictus Equilibrium

thousands of lives. And if you have a toothache, you definitely need to visit a dentist. But when you have a tooth removed, in most cases, you haven't eliminated the cause of the pain - you just removed the tooth. You fought the consequence. And pain in another tooth is just a matter of time.

In this book, I want to show you a deeper and at the same time simpler view of the course of most processes in your body. Most processes in our bodies have not yet been fully studied by science, but logic and basic knowledge of evolution provide many extraordinarily logical answers. And I would like to share with you my scientific-evolutionary-logical vision of tuning our body.

I named this book "Invictus Equilibrium. Immunity, Stress Resistance, and Long Life." Invictus translates from Latin as invincible, unconquered. Equilibrium translates from Latin as balance. And this book is actually permeated with the idea of searching for and forming an unshakable balance between body and mind.

Everything you read in this book is not medical advice. The purpose of this book is to give you a basic understanding of the main processes in your body and guide you toward their proper adjustment. There will be many simplifications in this book for easier comprehension. I am not responsible for your experiments on your own body. Perceive everything written in this book as interesting hypotheses that may work. Everything that will be written in this book works better if you incorporate it into your life very gradually and very carefully. Constantly observe your body. Even the smallest changes are noticeable if you listen to your body. It is always communicating with you and always gives you signals. You just need to interpret them correctly. Remember that the brain doesn't like rapid changes. And this is the first not-so-obvious thing: to change your body - change your brain. It controls everything. The whole world around you is only in your head!

Chapter 1
Why All This?

> *"There is no favorable wind for the one who does not know where to sail."*
>
> **Seneca**

This is the most fundamental question you need to ask yourself. What is the meaning of my life? Why do I really need to be healthy? I want to live a long time, for what? What is my mission in this life? To build a great company? To write a book? To raise wonderful children? To plant a forest? To conquer the highest peak? To fly to another planet (which is actually not that far off)? Do I just want to enjoy life? Or maybe I want to do all this together and then set myself another dozen goals?

In reality, nobody knows anything about the meaning of life (at least not yet). Everyone has their own. Perhaps our meaning of life lies in its search. But one thing can be said for sure: our inner world always reflects the outer world, and the outer reflects the inner. And if deep inside, our subconscious doesn't realize why we exist, it will, by all possible means, bring us closer to death. Interestingly, death should not be feared. It should be accepted. It's an inevitable process. It will definitely happen, and it's impossible to escape from it. We have all already lost in this game. And death is one of the things we cannot control. It's a given. The place where you were born, your parents, the genetic features of your body, the weather tomorrow, the thoughts and actions of other people - all these are things we cannot control. Therefore, control what you can control, and don't worry about the rest.

But it's impossible and unnecessary to completely get rid of fear. Fear should exist. And it's the fear of living this life in vain. Not utilizing all those opportunities that each of us has. Not fulfilling your mission. Not experiencing this life to the fullest. And for all this, it's worth fighting.

It is necessary to clearly realize that we are all unique and extraordinarily complex organisms. No one on this planet knows exactly how our body works, and especially our brain. We are all the greatest creation of nature and at the same time the biggest mystery of nature. And there is only one person on this planet who is capable of solving this mystery. And that is you yourself. You are unique. You are the only one on this

Invictus Equilibrium

planet who has found yourself in such a situation. Your life is as unique as possible, and no one but you can fully comprehend it.

No one but you will fight for your **Life**!!!

No one but you will fight for your **Happiness**!!!

No one but you will fight for your **Success**!!!

People die en masse,

but they save themselves individually!

Chapter 2

Evolution Is Killing You!

> *"A person has no meaning in life if they do not pay attention to their body and health."*
>
> **Abraham Maslow**

In fact, this is not just a loud headline. It's the absolute truth that is not customary to talk about. Today's world has greatly lulled most of us, and we all stop noticing how we are losing vital energy, control over our lives, and consequently life itself. And I will prove this to you and hope that you have enough strength to wake up.

Our civilization as a whole has progressed extraordinarily over the last few hundred years. Vaccines and antibiotics have been discovered; there has been a colossal development in surgery and other fields of medicine. Today, we all know a lot about hygiene, and most of the planet's population has access to clean drinking water. Most can access an infinite amount of information just by putting their hand in their pocket and taking out their phone. Many of us have become excellent masters of hunting for discounts in supermarkets and have completely forgotten the real feeling of hunger. And these are certainly not all the civilizational breakthroughs that have occurred in just the last 100 years. If you look at the average life expectancy in the world, over the past 100 years it has increased by 31 years (from 42 to 73 years)[1]. This is actually a colossal number and may seem like everything is much better than it could be. And there's some truth in this. But all of this has another side of the coin.

Over the last 150 years, the consumption of refined sugar per person has increased 50 times, leading to an obesity epidemic (visible to the naked eye), a sharp increase in people with type 2 diabetes, and cardiovascular diseases[2]. The level of testosterone in men over the last 120 years has decreased on average by 1.2% per year, and this trend is observed in all age groups. That is, in 1900, a 50-year-old had on average an order of magnitude more testosterone than a 20-year-old today[3]. And testosterone is not only about aggression, ambition, motivation, physical strength, and the like; it is, after all, the hormone directly responsible for reproductive function. Add to this the constant informational and noise load (especially in megacities), which creates constant psychological stress. As a result, the number of people with various mental disorders grows every year. And even this is enough to realize that progress does not always bring only benefits. And this is far from a complete list of not very useful things that modern times present us all. As certain studies show, there is a trend of decreasing real levels of happiness and life satisfaction among most young people compared to previous generations[4]. And the normal functioning of the body plays a significant role in all of this. Through rethinking and adjusting the normal operation of your body as a single system, you can change not only the world around you but also the world inside you, through the physical alteration of your set of genes. And here I am absolutely serious.

Your genome (the totality of all your genes) is like a set of blocks in a Lego construction set. This set is unique for everyone, but no one has an exact instruction on how to assemble it. Figuratively speaking, your body assembles this set based on the example of your parents, only starting from the end result. It's like building a house from a photograph of an already built house. It will turn out similar but not an exact copy. And by changing your habits and lifestyle, you can change this instruction and, as a result, rebuild your house. In this world, millions of the most diverse houses have been built, and most of them are constructed from absolutely

Invictus Equilibrium

identical building materials. Therefore, much depends on you in building your own strong house.

From all this, we can conclude that most of us use only a part of our real potential that our body and mind possess. The knowledge that I will highlight in this book allows you to really rethink life and change it. But only if you actually have such a need and, most importantly, the desire.

Chapter 3

Basics

"He who knows the cause controls the effect."

Folk Wisdom

Our body is a very complex mechanism where everything is connected to everything else. Even a small wound on your leg can cause headaches. It's not obvious, but a small wound on the leg makes you change your gait; as a result, blood circulation changes throughout your body, which can lead to insufficient blood flow in certain parts. And where there's not enough blood, various deficiencies begin to form, and consequently, problems start. This is a very primitive example, and I made it to help you understand that treating individual organs in our body without a comprehensive approach is very often not the right solution. Everything is interconnected. Problems in specific parts of the body are often a consequence, not the cause. They certainly need to be addressed because they already exist, but you also need to think about what led to them and how to avoid them. A healthy lifestyle is actually not about health. It's about the quality of life, about the ability to fill it with positive emotions. About the possibility of receiving brighter emotions that benefit the body and, as a result, prolong positive feelings.

Most people know that sugar and foods containing it are harmful to the body. In nature, there are no products with refined sugar (we're talking about pure sucrose, which as a chemical compound is found in fruits, but its effect on the body in this context is completely different because fruits contain a large number of nutrients that completely change the overall absorption process). Refined sugar is an absolutely unnatural product for us, but the amount of energy that sugar gives creates an explosion of pleasure in our minds, leaving a certain mark. But I can confidently say that most people on this planet have actually forgotten what it means to get real pleasure from sweets. Just imagine how a piece of festive cake would taste if you didn't eat sweets at all for a year. It would be an atomic explosion of pleasure that could be compared to many potent drugs but with minimal harm to the body (if you don't eat the whole cake yourself). This is the essence of balance and the relativity of being: creating conditions where the emotions you receive greatly outweigh potential harm. In my opinion, there's no point in giving up everything. There are simply things that are devoid of meaning. And it makes sense to understand the mechanisms of their action and, based on this knowledge, seek your own balance of emotions and health.

Comprehensive approaches to taking care of your health bring the best results. Of course, it's better to do at least something than nothing, but if you adjust your sleep and do not eat properly, the effect will not be significant. And no matter how well you eat and exercise, if you don't have normal sleep, the effect on your well-being will also be negligible or may even be negative. Therefore, your main task should be to find a balance of all these things in your life. Even stress, in small amounts, is extremely beneficial for our body. And to start understanding your body better, you need at least to delve a bit into the basic concepts: How does our body work? Why does it work this way? What affects our body? What is the logic of processes in our body? What signals does our body send us? And so on.

In fact, all our perception of the world is very conditional. Try to imagine how you would explain to a blind person how the color red differs from green. And now imagine how they would understand it. Not an easy task for the imagination. And considering that we are all very different, you need to test everything on yourself and track what really works well for you and what doesn't. What is beneficial for one person can be harmful to another. Therefore, everything you read in this book definitely works. But you should perceive all the information as a recommendation to try and derive your own formula for bulletproof health from all this knowledge.

Genetics and Epigenetics

This is not the easiest topic to grasp, but we need to start with it to truly make you understand that you can physically influence any process in your body. This can often be challenging, but the most important thing is to realize that it is actually possible. As Lao Tzu said: "The journey of a thousand miles begins with one step."

In general, genetics is the science that studies heredity and the ability of organisms to acquire new traits that differ from those of their ancestors. And this is the main thing to understand. Your genetic code is not static and can change during your life depending on the conditions you're in, although not so long ago scientists believed that changes in the genetic code were impossible. But a science like epigenetics tells us that mechanisms for controlling DNA sequences do exist, and our body actively uses them.

Epigenetics is the science that studies changes in gene expression strength that are not associated with actual changes in the DNA sequence. In simple terms, you have a set of genes, and there's a mechanism that can control the action of each individual gene without actually changing the DNA. That is, your body under different conditions can simply turn on or off a specific gene. Imagine you have a car, but if you've never started it and it just stands in your yard, its usefulness is zero. Conversely, if you're sitting on a broken chair, until you stop using it, it will bring you more harm than good. In terms of genetics, you can't throw away the chair, but you can simply stop using it. Interestingly, these epigenetic features can be inherited.

For example, there is a study that shows the correlation between a mother's nutrition during pregnancy and the propensity of her children, and even grandchildren, to obesity and cardiovascular diseases[1]. If a mother eats poorly during pregnancy, her descendants have an increased likelihood of obesity and various cardiovascular diseases. In another study, it was found that paternal grandfathers who experienced food shortages during puberty had grandchildren with a lower risk of diabetes and cardiovascular diseases. Conversely, grandfathers who ate excessively during puberty had grandchildren with an increased risk of diabetes and cardiovascular diseases[2].

Invictus Equilibrium

From all this, we can conclude that the conditions of our existence significantly affect our actual genome (through epigenetic mechanisms), and it can change throughout our lives. By changing your conditions, you can significantly affect your body and, consequently, your mind.

Hormones and Neurotransmitters

In simple terms, hormones and neurotransmitters are chemical substances that regulate absolutely all processes in our body. Their essence is the same; the names differ depending on where they are synthesized. If synthesized in the brain, they are neurotransmitters; if in glands, they are hormones. Need to wake up—a certain neurotransmitter is released into the blood; need to calm down—another is released, and so on. There is always some cocktail of hormones and neurotransmitters in our blood, and this completely forms our mood, well-being, ability to act, etc. There are many of them in our body; not all can be reliably measured, and not all can be influenced. But if you know the main ones, understand what reactions they cause in our body, and how you can influence their levels, you can significantly change your life.

Androgens – male sex hormones.

Estrogens – female sex hormones.

Dopamine – the "pleasure hormone" that is released at moments of pleasure and also during the anticipation of pleasure. Research shows that often the level during the anticipation stage is higher than during the pleasure itself (like expecting a win in a casino)[3]. It also plays a role in habit formation and motivation. Ate something delicious, exercised, completed your daily plan and praised yourself—you received a dopamine release as a reward. Similar in action to drugs like amphetamines.

Symptoms of dopamine deficiency include fatigue, memory problems, decreased concentration, trouble falling asleep and waking up, constant feelings of guilt, pessimistic mood, lack of desire to work, and the formation of dependencies on various stimulants and drugs.

With an excess, high levels of motivation, self-control, productivity, hyperactivity, feelings of satisfaction, and high libido are observed. A high level causes the body to be in constant stress; falling asleep and sleep in general worsen; it becomes impossible to relax.

Serotonin – responsible for mood formation (mainly feelings of joy and happiness), regulates muscle tone, affects memory, the learning process, feelings of reward, pain syndromes, and much more.

Invictus Equilibrium

Deficiency causes sharp mood swings, memory deterioration, sleep disturbances, increased aggression, decreased self-esteem, increased cravings for sweets and flour products, and feelings of unreasonable anxiety.

Excess leads to blood pressure spikes, coordination disorders, excitement and anxiety, rapid heartbeat, and possible loss of consciousness.

Testosterone – the main male sex hormone. Responsible for the development of genitals and secondary sexual characteristics. Directly affects the development of bone and muscle tissue, sexual behavior, and the manifestation of dominance. Testosterone levels in adult men are 15–20 times higher than in women.

Insufficient levels in men lead to infertility, development of mammary glands, loss of libido, manifestations of erectile dysfunction, general malaise, and lack of energy. With low levels, men exhibit a pronounced fear of competition, fear of confrontation, insecurity, fear of asserting themselves, and fear of responsibility.

At very high testosterone levels, hair loss on the head along with excessive body hair, excessive sweating, acne, voice changes, weight gain, and sharp mood swings are observed. In women, it manifests as irregular menstrual cycles.

Cortisol – the main stress hormone in the body. Synthesized from cholesterol that enters the body. Normally, the highest amount of cortisol is released in the morning to wake up the body, and its level gradually decreases throughout the day. It also affects brain function, supports the nervous system's performance, controls blood pressure, protects the body from infections, and regulates blood glucose levels.

Constant high cortisol levels can lead to decreased testosterone, fatigue, weakened immunity, muscle tissue breakdown, decreased bone strength, accumulation of fat deposits, sleep disturbances, accelerated heartbeat, aggression attacks, development of diabetes, and infertility.

With low cortisol levels, the development of liver cirrhosis and hepatitis, and adrenal gland disorders are possible.

Prolactin – responsible for breast formation and lactation in women, participates in forming maternal instincts, helps foster the desire to reproduce and raise offspring, and influences the formation of social bonds and tolerance toward others. It's intensively produced in women's bodies during pregnancy and breastfeeding.

With an excess in women, spontaneous milk secretion, absence of menstruation, possible headaches, and vision disturbances can occur. In men, excess weakens erection, reduces sexual desire, and may lead to breast enlargement of the female type.

At low levels in women, decreased libido, possible conception problems, headaches, psycho-emotional instability, and dizziness are observed. In men, possible depression, decreased libido, reduced sperm motility, and a tendency toward prostatitis.

Estradiol – the most active female sex hormone. Responsible for forming female secondary sexual characteristics and psychological features. Influences emotionality, mood swings, and the stability of the emotional state.

At high levels in women, excessive sweating, weight gain, appearance of various rashes, and hair loss are possible. In men, weight gain, baldness, and decreased sexual activity are observed.

At low levels in women, absence of menstruation, excessive skin dryness, sleep disturbances, irritability, mood swings, aggressiveness, and development of infertility are observed. In men, possible development of infertility, prostatitis, and cardiovascular diseases.

Melatonin – also called the "sleep hormone." A natural modulator of immunity. A natural sedative responsible for the speed of falling asleep, awakening, and the quality of sleep and body recovery during it.

With insufficient melatonin synthesis during sleep, high blood pressure, constant fatigue, lethargy, and loss of skin elasticity are possible; decreased sexual activity, frequent colds and infectious diseases, sleep disturbances, and possible weight gain are observed.

With excessive melatonin levels, dizziness, headaches, nausea, diarrhea, joint pain, irritability, increased daytime sleepiness, insomnia at night, and fluctuations in blood pressure are possible.

Adrenaline – strongly stimulates the nervous system, accelerating it in stressful situations. Under adrenaline, pulse increases, blood pressure rises, blood flow to muscles increases; at high levels, it reduces the feeling of pain. There are documented cases where completely untrained people

Invictus Equilibrium

lifted over 300 kg in stressful situations and didn't feel pain from muscle tears.

Deficiency can cause depression, mood swings, apathy, and weak reactions to stressful situations.

Excess can provoke cardiovascular diseases, tumor development, and rapid weight loss.

Noradrenaline – also called the "hormone of rage," responsible for brain activity, concentration, and memory.

With deficiencies, apathy, weakness, drowsiness, depressive states, frequent headaches, sadness, and muscle pain are possible.

With elevated levels, panic attacks, anxiety, blood pressure spikes, and problems with falling asleep are possible.

Gamma-Aminobutyric Acid (GABA) – the main inhibitory neurotransmitter in our brain. Reduces excitation and helps focus and calm down. Participates in controlling movements, attention, and emotions.

At low levels, the formation of various anxiety states, constant feelings of physical tension, periodic tremors, heavy sweating, inability to focus, problems with falling asleep due to nervousness, mood swings, mood and behavior disorders due to stress, feelings of fatigue, periodic breathing difficulties, confusion of thoughts, nervousness, inability to relax, and the development of epilepsy are possible.

Excessive levels lead to nausea, increased anxiety, fever, and shortness of breath.

Oxytocin – a hormone that causes feelings of satisfaction, reduced anxiety, and a sense of calm near a partner. Its role is to increase trust and reduce fear in human relationships. It inhibits cortisol release. Restores the brain's sensitivity to GABA when it's disturbed. Actively released during hugs and during sex. There's even the concept of a "hug deficit." It's proven that hugs reduce stress levels, improve heart health, boost immunity, increase happiness levels, help fight fears, and reduce feelings of pain—and I'm sure these aren't all the positive effects[4,5,6].

With deficiency, depressive states, depressed mood, anxiety disorders, development of schizophrenia, nervous system disorders, and menopause in women are possible.

Excess leads to general fatigue and poor adrenal gland function.

Immunity

Immunity is a complex multi-level system of built-in defense mechanisms in our body that detect foreign microorganisms and neutralize them. Approximately 80% of our immune system is located in our intestines in the form of lymphoid tissue, and from nature's point of view, this is quite logical. Most direct contacts of our body with various bacteria and viruses occur there. But need remember that almost all cells in our body have immune functions. There are central immune organs (thymus and bone marrow) and many secondary ones. Immunity always works and protects us from external (bacteria, viruses, fungi, toxins, etc.) and internal (infected and mutated cells) threats. Every day, our body gets rid of 45–65 billion defective cells. There's innate immunity (formed in the mother's womb) and acquired immunity (formed after encountering a new infection). There's also the concept of local and general immunity. For example, our skin has an immune function and almost always acts as the first barrier to any infection. If you have a wound on your body or dried mucous membranes, for example, the external barrier in those places will be weaker, making it easier for infections to enter the body. Therefore, simply humidifying the air in dry regions can often bring no less benefit than taking vitamins.

How does immunity work in general? Let's imagine a virus has entered our body. The innate immunity, in the form of neutrophils and macrophages, reacts first. The main task of neutrophils is to kill the unknown virus; they can also produce substances that attract other immune cells to the invading virus. These are suicide cells—they destroy the enemy and die (pus consists of dead neutrophils). Macrophages also consume viruses; they are larger, can work longer, and can introduce other immune cells to virus fragments so the body can fight it better.

In most cases, innate immunity is not enough, and acquired immunity begins to engage. Immunity has scouts in the form of dendritic cells that collect virus remnants, cover themselves with them, and go in search of specific T-cells. The dendritic cell selects a specific T-cell that matches a specific virus and can fight it. Then the dendritic cell activates the correct T-cell. All T-cells undergo immune training in the thymus (one of the main immune glands in the body). Then the properly trained T-cells begin to actively clone themselves. And then a bloody battle ensues, where different immune cells destroy all the viruses. As a result of this battle, our body produces antibodies to the specific virus and converts them into memory cells that carry information about this virus to protect our body during repeated attacks.

Invictus Equilibrium

Our body is super adaptive and can adjust, under favorable conditions, to almost anything. But there are a few points to pay attention to. There's the hygiene hypothesis, according to which children who get sick more often in childhood often have better immunity in adulthood than those who were rarely ill as children[7]. And there's logic to this.

To understand why this happens, we need to figure out how immunity is formed in a child. Immunity in a child up to one year old is almost absent and is highly dependent on the mother's immunity, which is transmitted to the child through breast milk. That's why breastfeeding is very important for a child in the first year. Between one and three years old, the first stage of immunity formation occurs. Then several more stages follow, and during puberty (13–15 years old), the last active period of immunity formation happens. After that, the formation of new immune experiences declines. If a child frequently contacts various pathogens until the end of the active period, it contributes to a more active and natural formation of the immune system, making it more versatile.

What conclusions should we draw from all this? The ideal childhood for our child will be when they eat well, sleep well, move a lot, constantly communicate with many other children (and animals), and come into contact with various new potential pathogens (getting sick 4–6 times a year is normal for a child; with a high level of immunity, most of these illnesses will pass asymptomatically or in a mild form). But this doesn't mean you need to infect your child with all possible diseases in turn. There are many diseases that are genuinely better never to contract, as irreversible changes in the body are possible after them. But if you see your child eating dirt, kissing your dog, and they're fine afterward, know that they're just exploring the world and training their immunity. For adults, the general health condition of the body is a more important factor. If you have symptoms of chronic fatigue, prolonged illnesses that occur without a fever, poorly healing wounds, presence of herpes or a large number of papillomas and warts, this may indicate a low level of immunity. The more vital energy you have and the higher your metabolic processes, the better and faster your body will cope with existing and new threats.

Chapter 4

The Brain

"Those who can transform themselves will transform the world, knowing that the greatest mastery begins with the control of the mind. When the mind becomes an obedient servant of a person, the whole world will lie at their feet."

Confucius

This is the most important thing to realize. Our entire life is in our heads. Everything you see, feel, hear - is what your brain has created for you. It completely controls your perception of this world and does so without your knowledge. For example, you hate tomatoes, and the moment you see them, you develop a gag reflex. But if you are not fed for 3–7 days and then given tomatoes, it turns out to be the most delicious thing you've ever eaten in your life. And so it is with everything.

Your brain will always adapt to the external environment and won't ask you. Absolutely everything that happens in your life changes your brain irreversibly. Everything that once gets into your head leaves its mark there forever. But if you understand a bit how and why it reacts to different situations, you can turn it in the direction you need and completely change your life. All changes begin in the head. But it's very important to know that the brain doesn't like rapid changes. If you try to break your supercomputer with very rapid changes, this can often lead to a worse result than before the changes began. There are plenty of heroic stories of people who incredibly quickly changed their lives in the direction they needed, but no one talks about the even greater number of those who ruined their lives. Therefore, you should find your own pace and constantly change in the direction of your goal. Even a mountain can be dismantled one small stone at a time.

Structure of the Brain

Our brain is a very complex system that has been forming for hundreds of millions of years, but if you have a basic understanding of the structure of our brain and comprehend it without illusions, you can understand where the brain is our friend and where it is our enemy. And it's worth starting with the fact that we are at least 90% animals.

Invictus Equilibrium

Our awareness of our existence is only a small part of what the brain shows us. Most processes in our body occur without our conscious participation and are fully programmed. No one can control how much gastric juice will be released during eating, how many beats the heart will make in the next minute, how many hours you will sleep, etc.

The existence of free will is still a complete mystery, and our animal nature is very easily demonstrated by an infinite number of simple experiments. Imagine a huge hammer and an anvil in front of you, and in a few seconds, the hammer will strike the anvil with great force and noise. You know for sure that the hammer will hit the anvil and it will be very loud, but try at that moment not to blink using your willpower. If you don't have psychological deviations and this is happening for the first time in your life, no matter how hard you try, you will always blink. And this will happen automatically. But if you work in an enterprise where there is constant such influence, your brain will rebuild, and you will no longer blink during the hits. That is, we can conclude that our present is programmed by our genes by 90% (and possibly 99%), and, no less importantly, by the environment. And if we gradually change the external influence on our body and brain, we can influence our future through the gradual formation of correct habits.

Regarding the physical structure, our brain is simplified into three main parts: the reptilian brain (R-complex), the limbic system, and the neocortex (cerebral cortex).

The **Reptilian Brain** is the brain that structurally resembles the brain of reptiles. It is the oldest part of our brain and was formed more than 100 million years ago. It is responsible for our basic behavior: breathing, movement, heartbeat, digestion, aggression, the instinct of reproduction, striving for hierarchy, struggle for power, the desire to control everything and own everything, protection of one's own territory, deception, stereotyped thinking, ritual behavior, and the like. This is the cold-blooded part of our brain; it does not think about other people or the consequences of our actions for them. The reptilian brain always reacts immediately to situations. It is our autopilot, based on simple reactions of "fight - freeze - flee." Its main task is to protect the body at any cost.

The **Limbic System** is our emotional brain. We inherited it from ancient mammals and it is 98% identical to their brain. Perhaps that is why we love animals so much. It is responsible for the instinct of self-preservation, self-defense, maternal care, upbringing, social behavior management, and the like. It is the main generator of emotions and connects physical activity with emotional. Psychotropic substances affect this part of our brain. It is important to understand that it does not like changes. It will strive with all its might for safety, comfort, and stability. Any attempts to leave the comfort zone are always stressful for it, and almost always, what you want is located beyond your comfort zone.

It does not distinguish between psychological and physical threats. That is why verbal disputes very easily turn into fights. If it is attacked, even with words, it defends itself.

This brain is focused on the moment "now." For it, there is no future. It transfers all feelings from the past as if it's all happening now and repeats the emotional state. If you once fell from a tree, then every subsequent situation associated with height will cause emotions similar to the first until the brain realizes otherwise through multiple positive experiences. And here it makes sense to write a bit about learned helplessness, because the formation of this psychological state is strongly connected with the limbic system and is quite common today.

Learned helplessness is a psychological state in which a person (or animal) believes that there is no control over the situation and therefore does not try to change it even when the possibility for change appears. It often forms after a person has experienced uncontrollable adverse situations, after which a feeling of powerlessness is formed. This phenomenon was first described by Martin Seligman in the 1960s. In his experiments, he took several dogs and placed them in boxes where the dogs were given mild electric shocks. Some dogs had the ability to counteract the electric shocks, while others did not. And after the dogs without the ability to influence the shocks stopped actively reacting to the situation, they were given the opportunity to turn off the electric current, but even in this case, they did not start using it because they were already completely disillusioned with the possibility of changing anything and simply endured painful sensations.

It was important to write about this effect because the strength of psychological effects decreases significantly when their action becomes known. And there are studies that demonstrate this well[1]. It's not so easy to hypnotize a hypnotist, especially if he doesn't want it.

The **Cerebral Cortex** is our most rational brain. It is the youngest. It is about 2.5 million years old. This is what we are used to calling the mind. All our thoughts, processes of cognition, and analysis occur in it. It occupies most of the skull. It has about 15 trillion neurons and 10 with 13 zeros neural connections. Just imagine that in your head alone, the number of different possible combinations of all these connections is greater than the number of all electrons and

Invictus Equilibrium

protons in our Universe. If you try to write down this number, it would take 75 years to write the zeros. This makes our brain an extraordinary thinking machine. Each of us has about 60,000 different thoughts per day.

One might think that our brain is extremely conscious, but about 98% of processes occur subconsciously. Paul MacLean said: "We must look at ourselves and the world through the eyes of three completely different personalities, two of which are unarmed with language."

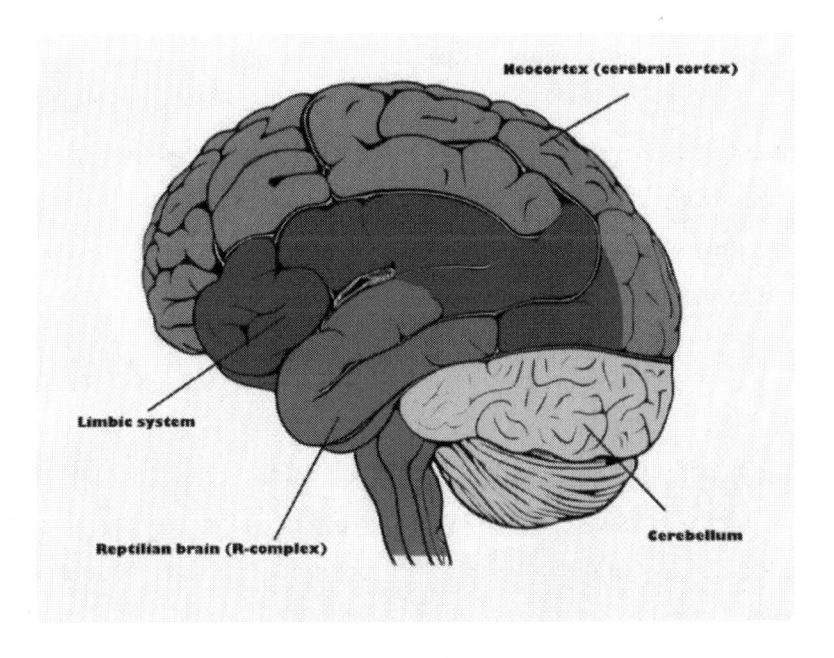

A schematic representation of the division of our brain into parts

Neuroplasticity

Since our brain subconsciously controls almost everything, it makes sense to figure out whether we can at least slightly influence these processes and their course. And here we need to mention neuroplasticity.

Neuroplasticity is the ability of our brain to physically change its structure and functions in response to certain stimuli (damage, learning, acquisition of new experiences). This phenomenon was first noticed by various scientists back in the 19th century, and since then it has been confirmed by a huge number of various studies. Neuroplasticity shows that our nervous system is extremely flexible and can adapt to any conditions. Thanks to neuroplasticity, the brain can change existing neural connections, form new ones, and even restore lost functions.

The main features of neuroplasticity are the brain's ability to neurogenesis (the ability of the brain to form new neurons, which is directly related to learning and memory), synaptic plasticity (the brain can physically change the strength of connections between neurons, which is the basis of memory and the learning process), and reorganization of neural networks (the brain can redistribute certain functions between different areas, which is well seen in the adaptations of people during recovery after severe head injuries or after the loss of certain functions, like hearing, when in the deaf the ability for tactile sensations and similar increases significantly).

It is clear that every brain and organism as a whole has certain natural limitations on the potential peak of capabilities. Everyone will develop at different speeds. But the main thing is that the ability for potential development is built into every body and mind by nature. And no one knows exactly where the peak of their personal capabilities actually is. The fact that you are developing slowly at the beginning does not mean that it will always be so. Therefore, regardless of the speed at which you are developing today and the point you are at, know that a well-built regime (sleep, nutrition, physical activity, stress control, and the like) can greatly affect your potential development capabilities.

Forming Habits

If your life is monotonous, and you constantly watch series, spend time on social networks, or play games instead of doing something useful, then you're not lazy. You're just very disciplined.

Our brain doesn't like changes and will always try to stay in comfortable and, more importantly, familiar conditions for it. And from a biological point of view, today, for most people, conditions are very comfortable. Most people on this planet eat more than once a day; we have homes, a bunch of cheap dopamine in the form of TV shows, social networks, etc. Therefore, our brain doesn't perceive any changes very joyfully. And that's why the idea of changing all your habits in one day, which have been forming for many, many years, is not very good.

So how do you form new habits? First, you should realize that your habits will stay with you forever. You only have the option to form new ones so that your brain has no desire to return to the old ones. You need to create conditions in which your brain will understand that new habits are more priority than old ones. Know that if you overdo it in forming new habits, your brain can easily convince you that your new habits are something very bad. Radicalism won't benefit most people and can only harm. Taking one step back to then take two steps forward is a normal story.

For example, you want to start running. If you're untrained and run 10 kilometers (6.21 miles) in the first training and barely make it home half-alive, your brain will make a very simple conclusion: "Went for a run. Almost died. Running is deadly dangerous. Shouldn't run anymore." But if you run 300 meters (328 yards), your brain will have a different conclusion: "Went for a run. Pulse slightly increased. Nothing terrible happened. Received a small portion of dopamine because I ran more than planned (since I planned to run 100 meters (109 yards))." And if you do this many times, the neural connections in your brain will form so strong that you won't need to make volitional efforts to run. And then you can transform this habit as you wish. Even very hard workouts won't create a desire to stop.

In forming new habits, planning and highlighting completed tasks also help a lot. If you simply write down your small tasks for the day in a notebook and put checkmarks next to them upon completion, this will cause dopamine releases in your head and emphasize the necessity of these tasks. Even a very small victory is still a victory. Set big goals for yourself, but always break them down into many small ones that can be quickly completed. It's simpler for the body and mind.

There are a lot of different data on the time it takes to form a habit. But we are all so different that it's simply impossible to calculate the exact number of days. According to a study by scientists from University College London, a habit can form from 18 to 254 days (the average number of days is 66)[2]. I think you can even find a very small percentage of people for whom some habits won't form even after 300 days. The speed of formation also strongly depends on which habit you want to form. Simple habits form faster (just drinking water in the morning), complex ones take longer (exercising 3 times a week in the gym for 45 minutes). The main thing is to understand that forming a new habit is not always a quick process and just not to stop on the way to the set goal.

What should be understood? Any habit is essentially a ritual. Any habit has actions that precede it and that the brain remembers and associates. If you don't have games on your work phone, then when you take it in your hands, your brain launches the "work" program in your head because it doesn't associate this phone with games since you've never played games on it. But if you start playing games on your work phone, your brain will begin to associate it with games, not with work. Therefore, it is very important to separate processes from each other. If you work in bed and sleep in bed, you end up with poorly done work and poor sleep. Everything should have its own place and its own ritual. If you buy separate running shoes and a sports suit for running, then already when you put them on, your brain will launch the running program. For example, today you have a planned run of 300 meters (328 yards), but you really don't feel like running today. That's normal. There are times when it's very hard to force yourself to do something. In such a situation,

Invictus Equilibrium

you should just start performing the ritual. Agree with yourself that today you'll just put on your suit and shoes and sit for 2 minutes in the hallway. After starting the ritual, it will be much easier to agree with yourself on a 100-meter (109 yards) run around the house. This works in reverse as well. To get rid of a bad ritual, you should identify its triggers and gradually eliminate them. If you physically don't have sweets at home, it will be hard to overeat them.

    I also believe that when forming a new habit, the most important thing is internal conviction for forming the habit. Sincerely convince yourself why you need the new habit. Also, don't forget that any new habit is stress. And in fact, forming a new habit is training your body and brain to process new stress. Stress is quite beneficial for the body, but in small amounts. Try not to allow prolonged high levels of cortisol in your body. Therefore, the most effective way to form new habits is to very gradually introduce them into your life. It's very important not to break yourself. Someone can introduce 3 new habits a week simultaneously, while for someone else, 1 a month is a lot. Don't forget to listen to yourself. Planned to run 300 meters (328 yards), but feel the strength to run a kilometer (1,093 yards). Then do it! Planned 3 km, but after the first one, you feel something's wrong. There's nothing bad about having a short workout. The main thing is to do it. You didn't run at all yesterday.

Also, our brain does not perceive attempts. You are not trying to start running. You are running. You are already a runner. You are not trying to lose weight. You are losing weight. What you truly convince yourself of—that will become your reality. Self-suggestion works, and there are studies that prove it[3]. If you really believe in what you're doing, sincerely believe that you will actually succeed, and move toward the set goal, your strength multiplies many times over. And Kurt Richter's experiments perfectly demonstrate the effect of self-belief. He took rats, placed them in a container of water, and waited until they drowned. The average time of their struggle until death was 15 minutes. But when, at the moment of drowning, Kurt pulled the rats out, let them dry and regain strength, the next time they held on in the water for up to 80 hours, which reasonably suggests that the hope of rescue gave them an incredible amount of strength[4].

Evolution of Mass Dumbing Down

All people are extremely curious. Each of us is extremely greedy for information, and our brain is very bad at separating good from bad. It wants to know everything. It always rewards us with dopamine when receiving information. And this is our evolutionary adaptation. Millions of years ago, when our ancestors lived in savannas, fields, and forests, any information was extremely important. If a leaf

Invictus Equilibrium

rustled near you and you didn't pay attention, it could cost you your life. You could simply be eaten by a tiger. And today, marketing very skillfully uses this evolutionary adaptation of ours, and hooks us all on various dopamine needles.

Everything around us is surrounded by colorful banners and bright advertising. Social networks are filled with sexualized or violent content, including news. Computer games, pornography, fights, movies, and TV series—all this greatly exhausts our psyche, steals our energy and ability to concentrate, can cause addictions, and really significantly changes our brain. All these things just want to take all your time, and they succeed. Teenagers spend an average of 7.5 hours a day on media[5]. And even if you don't take into account studies that actually prove the formation of addictions to all these things through physical changes in the brain, how can this be logically explained if not as an addiction? A person spends 7.5 hours on something that only creates the illusion of benefit, but in most cases, actually carries nothing (just try to remember what videos you watched three days ago). And these are not just horror stories. This is science and statistics. And as the life experience of many people shows, those who already have one addiction more easily form another, and layering one addiction on another almost always leads to a complete loss of control over oneself and one's life.

The trouble is that our brain perceives all this flow of information as useful for us. It is important for us to know what is happening in the neighboring tribe (news), how to interact in society (TV series), who is the strongest male (fights), etc. Is it possible to refuse all this in today's world? Probably not completely (movies can be good). But all this definitely needs to start being controlled if you don't aim to degenerate completely.

There is an interesting experiment. Three similar groups of students are taken and given tests to solve. In the first group, each person's personal phone lies on the table; in the second group, the phone is in the pocket; in the third group, the phones are taken away, and they are in the room without them. As a result, the second group, with phones in their pockets, solves tests better than the first group, and the third group solves tests better than all. If everyone is swapped, the results do not change. Those whose phone is on the table solve tests the worst, and those who don't have a phone at all solve tests the best. It turns out that just the presence of a phone already significantly affects us. It makes us think about it and actually takes away part of our brain's power. The phone, in the literal sense, makes us dumber[6].

Our brain is super lazy and adaptive. If it can delegate some tasks to someone else, it will definitely do so. It gets

Invictus Equilibrium

used to the fact that all the world's problems can be solved by a simple box in your pocket and simply stops thinking and remembering anything. Also, the phone is often associated by our brain as a source of cheap dopamine. All this completely changes the structure of our brain. And it's scary. There are a lot of studies based on huge amounts of data in different countries that show that since the early 1980s, creativity in children has been constantly declining, the level of working memory is constantly declining, and the overall level of intelligence is also declining. And all this happens in clear correlation with the development of television and the internet. Paradoxically, the more technology develops, the more society as a whole becomes dumber[7,8].

So how to tame the endless flow of information that constantly pours onto your head? The most effective method is to limit the ability to absorb information. If you delete a social network, it will be hard for you to spend time on it. Find all the places where you lose your energy and time and just gradually get rid of them. Completely abandoning, for example, a smartphone in the current world is unlikely, but you can always find options for normal coexistence.

It is proven that smartphones really cause addiction, which leads to the development of depression, deterioration of sleep, memory, and the like, and this is definitely worth realizing[9,10,11]. All app developers are fighting for your attention and use many unfair (but still legal) methods to capture it. Like it or not, but inside we are a bit animals, and they are very skillful in using this. Therefore, first, you should realize your addiction (just look at your screen time on your phone, and everything will be clear) and then start using the same unfair methods in fighting it. Ask yourself whether you really need a smartphone or maybe you can get by with the simplest button phone (like the old NOKIA 3310). If you still decide that you need a smartphone, then start by turning off all possible notifications and allocate, for example, an hour in the evening to check mail, social networks, etc. Stop using it constantly and reduce its impact and importance for your brain. Track what things can steal your focus. For example, you took out your phone to check the time and started browsing social networks, even though you didn't plan to. A similar story is possible with an alarm clock. Track these moments, and maybe it makes sense to buy a regular watch and alarm clock. You can set time limits for specific apps or the entire smartphone. Don't sit on your smartphone constantly if it's not related to your work. Setting a black-and-white screen mode on your phone helps a lot in reducing screen time. Don't forget that we are all animals, and different colors excite our nervous system in very different ways. And marketers know this very well. And when there are no colors,

Invictus Equilibrium

it's harder to capture your attention. Try it. It will save you a lot of time, increase your productivity and concentration.

How to find energy, overcome procrastination, and start doing something? First, it's worth understanding that our brain cannot sit idle, and it always needs to be doing something. The desire to sit on the phone instead of working is not rest but simply the desire of our brain to replace a less pleasant activity with a more pleasant one in its understanding at the moment. And if you find yourself in a situation where you don't want to do anything, you simply have no strength for work, and it needs to be done, then the best option is to do nothing. Just lie down on the couch (I also like lying on the floor) and look at the ceiling. If you're really tired, you'll just fall asleep, and there's nothing wrong with that. But if your brain is just procrastinating, then after some time of staring at the ceiling, you will have a genuine desire to do something. Boredom is the strongest motivator. Even the most uninteresting work is more interesting than boredom. Realize that sitting on the phone, watching TV series, and the like is not rest. All this steals your vital energy, literally makes you dumb, and distracts you from really important things in your life. Therefore, you need to start treating all this very seriously and radically control the influence of these things on your brain.

Chapter 5

Sleep

"Sleep is the golden chain that connects our body and mind."

Thomas Dekker

Adjusting your sleep schedule is the first thing you need to do to build strong health. Poor sleep can disrupt any process in your body. No matter how much you exercise, how well you eat, or how many vitamins you consume, if you have poor sleep, the effectiveness of all your efforts to change something in your life will decrease many times over.

Studies on mice show that lack of sleep leads to a decrease in the number of immune cells, physical reduction of the brain, sharp weight loss (weight decreases despite an increase in calorie intake), and much more. The ultimate result of sleep deprivation in mice is sudden death[1,2,3,4]. Similar experiments are not conducted on humans, but there are studies on partial sleep deprivation.

Systematic insufficient sleep leads to an increased risk of mortality, a higher incidence of cardiovascular diseases, increased risk of type 2 diabetes, decreased cognitive abilities with a growing risk of cognitive impairments, a significant increase in the risk of obesity, elevated levels of stress hormones in the blood, worsened memory and immune responses, a higher likelihood of accidents and workplace injuries, and much more[5,6,7]. According to American scientists, in the U.S. alone, at least 1,500 people die each year due to sleep deprivation, often in car accidents caused by drowsy driving.

There is also data indicating that excessive sleep duration is associated with increased mortality risk, occurrence of cardiovascular diseases, and other negative effects[5]. However, my personal opinion is that insufficient sleep is the cause of problems, while increased sleep duration in most cases is a consequence of existing issues and the body's attempt to solve these problems through extended sleep.

When it comes to sleep in general, we actually know almost nothing about it. What is sleep? Why do we need it? How did it evolve? All these are open questions. From an evolutionary standpoint, sleep is absolutely disadvantageous for us because during sleep we are completely defenseless, increasing the likelihood of being preyed upon. However, there are several partially confirmed hypotheses about why we need sleep. During sleep, the accumulated information of the day is processed (unnecessary data is deleted and necessary information is structured), the body recovers, and sleep is extremely important for the proper development of the brain in children. Additionally, night is an inefficient time for us, so the body tries to conserve energy. There is also a hypothesis that during the day, the brain processes information received from the outside (through sight, smell, etc.), and at night it processes information from internal organs, thereby diagnosing the body and solving internal problems.

During sleep, new neural connections are formed, but the brain processes everything that happened during the day from the end to the beginning. Therefore, information you study before sleep is remembered better than what you learn in the morning. Studies on mice show that the brain replays everything that happened during the day during sleep and decides what needs to be retained and what should be discarded[8].

The quality of sleep in our body is regulated by the hormone melatonin. The amount synthesized directly depends on the amount of light that reaches our retinas. Even when

Invictus Equilibrium

your eyes are closed, your brain clearly understands whether it is day or night. Evolutionarily, this mechanism is easy to explain. As soon as the sun begins to set, the amount of light decreases, and the brain starts preparing for sleep. When the sun rises, the amount of light increases, and the body awakens. Therefore, to ensure high-quality sleep, you need to sleep in a completely dark room. This can be achieved by using a sleep mask or blackout curtains. Complete darkness is truly one of the most important components of healthy sleep. Conversely, to wake up properly, you need bright light. If you often have to wake up at night, shining a bright lamp into your eyes for a few minutes is a good idea (a practice used by submariners).

There are many charts suggesting that sleep efficiency is high at certain times and low at others, recommending that you go to bed at a specific hour. Personally, I think this is nonsense. Your body doesn't know what time it is and relies on specific processes within your body (mainly revolving around the amount of light). Everyone can create their own biorhythms. Try to go to bed at the same time each night, but it's better to wake up without an alarm clock; your body knows how much time it needs to recover. Research shows that the average duration of healthy sleep for most adults is between 7 and 8 hours. Less than that can lead to negative effects[5]. From personal experience, I can say that on days with a lot of physical work, you sleep a bit longer. If you can't get enough sleep time, it's better to use a smart alarm clock rather than a regular one. Our sleep is divided into four phases, and waking up during specific phases is less stressful for our body.

Sleep is not an instantaneous process. Our body gradually immerses itself into it. In today's world, we are surrounded by a lot of flickering blue light (from screens of various devices). To simplify, there is warm light (less bright) and cold light (brighter). Any cold light excites our nervous system (our brain perceives it as sunlight), so ideally, its exposure should be completely limited an hour or two before sleep to signal to our brain that the day has ended. There are many programs that adjust the warmth of your device screens before bedtime. But the best option is to avoid looking at screens before sleep altogether. For example, I read for an hour before bedtime, combining the useful with the beneficial. It's also better to replace all lighting in your home from cold to warm light. Evolutionarily, before sleep, the only light we could see was from fire, which is quite dim and warm.

Stimulants like nicotine, caffeine, and alcohol negatively affect sleep quality. They should not be consumed 4–6 hours before bedtime. Ideally, they should not be consumed at all (more on this later). Eating is also better done

Invictus Equilibrium

4 hours before sleep. There's a myth that coffee helps you wake up well. In reality, it doesn't work quite that way. We have a built-in awakening mechanism, and immediately after sleep, our cortisol levels rise to wake up the body. If you drink coffee immediately after waking up, it blocks the action of cortisol. Coffee has the best effect if you drink it 1–2 hours after waking. Regarding exercise, it improves sleep quality but only if not done right before bedtime. There should be at least 2, preferably 4 hours between exercise and sleep because physical activity significantly stimulates the nervous system, which needs time to calm down.

There's another interesting proven effect for improving sleep quality: sleeping under a heavy blanket. From what I understand, it's not suitable for everyone, and nuances should be considered. Sleeping under a heavy blanket reduces anxiety levels in people who already have high anxiety, can decrease insomnia, and alleviate symptoms of fatigue[9,10]. For most healthy people, using a heavy blanket will have almost no effect. However, it's worth noting that there are rare cases of sleep worsening (1 person out of 120 studied)[10]. The effect on children is also ambiguous, although parents report positive changes in their children's behavior.

This effect is specific, but it's worth mentioning because in some cases it works very well. It's also important to know that when choosing such a blanket, it should not be heavier than 10% of your body weight. In the studies I mentioned, 6 kg and 8 kg blankets were used.

In summary, if you decide to adjust your sleep and can't fall asleep at the time you've planned, it's easier to start falling asleep at the necessary time if you haven't been sleeping well for a few days prior. If you want to sleep, any time is a good time for sleep.

Chapter 6
Earth

"Gravity not only keeps us on Earth but also creates the foundation of our being."

Albert Einstein

In 1976, the Japanese scientist Kyoichi Nakagawa published an article titled "Magnetic Field Deficiency Syndrome and Magnetic Treatment." In it, he wrote about the results of 20 years of research on the impact of the Earth's magnetic field on the human body.

It has been scientifically proven that our body, due to the movement of fluids within it, creates a small magnetic field around us, which constantly coexists with the external magnetic field. According to the article, over many millions of years, our body has adapted to the Earth's magnetic field, and now it is a necessary component of our normal existence.

However, in today's world, there are many factors that can reduce the influence of the Earth's magnetic field on our body. The vast amount of iron and concrete around us shields us from the natural magnetic field and significantly reduces its impact. If our body frequently resides in an environment with a diminished magnetic field, this can lead to the so-called "Magnetic Field Deficiency Syndrome" in humans.

Manifestations of the "Magnetic Field Deficiency Syndrome" include headaches, poor sleep, general weakness, cardiovascular diseases, increased fatigue, stomach disorders, decreased work capacity, and a number of other symptoms. Symptoms of this syndrome appear without objective reasons—for example, insomnia and headaches that are very difficult to treat but respond well to changes in the magnetic field (there is a type of treatment known as magnetotherapy).

Personally, I do not fully understand how to relate to this information. There are simply no representative studies. Nakagawa's research is essentially the only one, at least from what I have found. If we look at this issue from the standpoint of logic and evolution, it is quite logical that our body has adapted to absolutely every influence, and it's impossible to say that the Earth's magnetic field does not affect us at all. We can say with certainty that when solar flares occur, which briefly and sharply affect the Earth's magnetic field, a large

Invictus Equilibrium

portion of people definitely feel it. There is also data indicating that the influence of the magnetic field decreases quite significantly in high-rise buildings. The higher the floor, the lower the level of the magnetic field due to multi-layered shielding. If we believe the data I once saw, above the 5th floor there is already a significant difference compared to measurements on the ground. Personally, I do not have long-term experience living above the 2nd floor, so based on personal feelings, I can't say much.

What are the solutions if you have symptoms of "Magnetic Field Deficiency Syndrome"? The best option is to try not to live, at least for some time, in a big city where there is significant shielding from iron-concrete structures. If that's not an option, try living closer to the ground and observe possible reactions of your body. As I already mentioned, above the 5th floor there is a significant difference in the strength of the magnetic field compared to the Earth's surface. Another option is magnetotherapy. On the internet, there are many different magnetic bracelets and similar items for magnetotherapy, which are quite inexpensive and may work. According to data from Nakagawa's article, the use of magnets is quite safe. Almost no side effects were detected even with a fivefold increase in magnetic exposure over the conventional therapeutic dose. Only 4 out of 166 people who participated in the study complained of a "dizzy" feeling in the head, which may be associated with improved blood circulation. Therefore, a small magnetic influence should not harm you in any way. However, I would still rely on internal sensations.

It's also worth noting that the article describes an interesting effect of the body's adaptation to the magnetic field. In patients who experienced noticeable improvements in well-being from magnetotherapy, the positive effects could disappear over a long period of constant use. That is, if you, for example, started wearing a magnetic bracelet and after a few weeks your headaches really stopped or your sleep improved, then it's worth stopping the use of the bracelet until the symptoms reappear. If you don't do this, the symptoms may return after approximately 6–8 months.

Such studies look very ambiguous, but as general statistics show, the more our society moves away from the evolutionarily natural environment for us, the more problems we get with our bodies.

Chapter 7
The Sun

"Only the Sun is capable

of creating new life

on Earth every day."

Leonardo da Vinci

The Sun is essential for life on our planet. It not only provides strength and energy to all living things but can also mercilessly take away strength and energy. We cannot exist without it, yet we also cannot be exposed to it constantly. It embodies both life and death in one package. In this sense, the Sun perfectly reflects the essence of our entire life and the presence of balance in the Universe. Everything can be a remedy, and everything can be harmful. Life always borders on death, and the Sun is perhaps the most vivid example of this.

The absence of sunlight in our lives negatively affects the overall health of our bodies. Conversely, an excess of sun exposure can literally kill us. When we are under the Sun, our brain synthesizes the neurotransmitter serotonin, which significantly influences our overall mood. But the Sun is not as benevolent as it might seem at first glance. It is well-established that prolonged sun exposure on the skin significantly increases the likelihood of developing various skin cancers. It also accelerates the aging process of the skin. If we recall tanning beds, they are prohibited for use under the age of 18 and not recommended up to the age of 35. I would not recommend using them at all. However, returning to the Sun, we still need to be exposed to it, but the optimal amount is very blurred and individual for each person.

The impact of ultraviolet (UV) radiation on the body greatly depends on skin color. The lighter the skin, the greater the effect of the Sun and the higher the likelihood of burns with prolonged exposure. The intensity of UV radiation is also significantly influenced by how far you live from the equator. The closer you are to the poles, the less intense the solar radiation. This is due to the angle at which the Sun's rays strike the Earth. At a right angle, the Sun's rays are the most harmful. Therefore, it's advisable to avoid the Sun in the middle of the day, especially if you live in warm regions and have very fair skin. It's better to take sunbaths in the morning and closer to the evening when the Sun's rays are less aggressive. Nowadays, it's very convenient to track the intensity of UV radiation through the Ultraviolet Index (UV Index), which is available in many weather applications. Anything above 3 out of 10 units requires you to think about skin protection. If the index is above 7, I would recommend anyone to avoid prolonged sun exposure.

An important aspect of sun exposure is the synthesis of vitamin D in our bodies as a result of UV rays acting on our skin. Vitamin D can also enter our bodies through food. There are many various studies measuring vitamin D levels in different regions of the planet; they differ slightly, but overall, we can conclude that more than half of the Earth's population either has a current deficiency of vitamin D or is very close to deficient values. This especially concerns people living more than approximately 4,000 km (about 2,500 miles) from the equator (roughly speaking, outside the latitudes of Africa). From an evolutionary point of view, this seems like true because today, most people actually spend little time in the Sun compared to our ancestors. Also, the vitamin and micronutrient content of today's food leaves much to be desired. However, it's worth noting that, statistically, in countries with the least deficiency of vitamin D (we're talking about sunny countries), there's the highest number of people with skin cancer. Therefore, it's important to be cautious with the Sun.

In general, vitamin D is extremely important for our bodies. Its deficiency disrupts many processes within us. It significantly affects the functioning of the immune and nervous systems, enhances mood, and reduces anxiety and depression. With a vitamin D deficiency, our bodies handle illnesses much worse, the likelihood of developing various cancers increases, and mortality among people who already have cancer rises. Calcium absorption by the body worsens, leading to various musculoskeletal diseases. The risk of developing diabetes and various cardiovascular diseases increases, and this is not the entire list. Also, those who do not have a vitamin D deficiency lose excess weight more easily.

So where can we get this much-needed vitamin D? First, it's important to note that vitamin D has two main forms: D_2 and D_3. D_2 can only enter our bodies through food, while D3 is synthesized in our bodies under the influence of UV radiation from the Sun's rays and is also found in animal products. Vitamin D_3 is considered more stable and is therefore more necessary for our bodies. Sources of vitamin D_3 include salmon, tuna, trout, eggs, sardines, cod liver oil, and red meat. Vitamin D_2 is present in products that spend a lot of time in the Sun, primarily various grains and mushrooms. However, in reality, to get a sufficient amount of vitamin D from food, you'd need half of your daily diet to consist of fish, which is definitely not suitable for everyone. Therefore, we definitely can't do without the Sun, and we shouldn't forget about dietary supplements either.

Regarding synthetic vitamin D, research shows that it is absorbed no worse than natural vitamin D (provided that it's a high-quality synthetic vitamin D). This seems plausible because, from what I know, in most cases, the raw materials for obtaining various forms of vitamin D are natural components. It's also worth noting that there are different forms of vitamin D, and it's hard to determine which is better. Everyone should choose an option that suits them. However, in most cases, vitamin D is absorbed less effectively on its own, so personally, I take it in a complex with D_3 + K_2. The absorption of vitamin D is also improved by zinc, magnesium, boron, and vitamin A. The recommended norm for adults is considered to be 800–2,000 IU, and for children up to 1,000 IU. Vitamin D has a cumulative effect in our bodies, so it's quite difficult to harm yourself with small dosages. Personally, I take it without a doctor's prescription during the winter period in the amount of 2,000 IU. The ideal option is periodic testing for vitamin D and selecting dosages based on specific numbers.

We should also mention sunscreen creams, and here it's not very complicated. To have sufficient protection, use creams with an SPF rating higher than 30. But it's also important to understand that when using sunscreen, vitamin D is not synthesized in our bodies.

With sunglasses, it's a bit more complicated. It's very important that they are of high quality. The main function of sunglasses is protection from UV radiation. If you wear glasses that are simply tinted but offer no UV protection, your pupils dilate because less light reaches them, and as a result, they receive increased harm from the higher amount of UV that reaches them. Therefore, choosing an accessory like sunglasses should be approached very seriously. Adequate protection is provided by glasses with a UV rating of at least 400. It's also quite important that they protect the eyes from all sides. Additionally, it's worth mentioning that, in general, our eyes have a protective mechanism against UV radiation in the form of a pigmented membrane consisting of layers of melanin. This protection begins to work actively after 20–30 minutes of being in the Sun.

Chapter 8
Water

"Pure water is the first and most important doctor for the body and soul."

Sebastian Kneipp

Our bodies are composed of approximately 70% water, so it's safe to say that water is one of the most important elements of our existence. It is an extremely mysterious compound. No one understands where it came from on our planet and why we have so much of it (75% of our planet's surface is covered with water). To this day, there's no definitive answer as to why ice is slippery while other liquids in solid form are not. It is the only liquid known to us in which the density decreases when it transitions to a solid state (ice floats on water rather than sinking), which allows living organisms in freezing bodies of water to survive because they almost never freeze completely thanks to this property. In general, water has 18 already identified varieties of ice and at least 64 properties that distinguish it from all other known liquids. Water is an incredible liquid that can both heal us and easily harm us.

Structure of Water

This may sound strange, but there are studies that claim water has "memory" and changes its structure depending on what happens around it. Water reacts to the emotional background surrounding it and alters its structure. This effect was first discovered by the Japanese researcher Masaru Emoto. He took a small amount of water and played different types of music near it or spoke various words. Then he shock-froze the water and examined the ice crystals that formed. Water that was exposed to positive influences (kind words, pleasant calm music) had symmetrical and beautiful ice crystals. Water that was subjected to negative influences (rock music, swear words) had asymmetrical and ugly ice crystals.

And everything seems wonderful here. Several books were written, many different pictures of ice crystals were produced, but the scientific community considers Masaru Emoto a pseudoscientist, and his experiments unreliable. In reality, I found only two studies that seemingly confirm Masaru Emoto's hypothesis, but they are also very

Invictus Equilibrium

questionable. The samples are small, and the experiments themselves raise questions. Most importantly, it's unclear what impact "properly" structured water has on our bodies. One study indicated that plants watered with "proper" water grow slightly better, but the sample size is very small.

If we consider this issue logically, I cannot confidently say that this effect does not work. Structure is very important. For example, let's take the chemical element C (carbon). Graphite is pure carbon, and diamond is pure carbon. The element is the same, but the graphite in your pencil is very soft, while diamond is extremely hard. And it's all because they have different structures. We can certainly say that our world is hundreds of times more complex than we currently think and know. There are an enormous number of different things and effects that do not yet align with the views of classical science and which cannot yet be explained. In fact, all our science is based on guesses and assumptions because all scientific theories begin with the words "let's assume that...". In my opinion, our society will not be able to comprehend the essence of all the processes surrounding us for a very long time, if ever. But we can say with certainty that in the long term, positive emotions affect us better than negative ones.

It's also worth mentioning a very interesting effect. There are studies showing that cows produce more milk if they are regularly played music by Mozart or Beethoven on the farm. The fat content also increases slightly[1]. It is clear that this is not exactly about the "memory" of milk but more about the emotional state of the cows, but why couldn't something similar work with water? Could it be that our internal state affects how well we absorb the water we drink?

Amount of Water

There are many opinions on how much water one should drink. The World Health Organization recommends drinking at least 30 ml of water per kilogram of body weight per day for an adult (1.01 US fl oz for 2.2 pounds). In general, this figure is close to accurate, but it's also important to understand that we are all different, and this number should be used as a guideline rather than an absolute value. Also, if you have a lot of excess weight, it's better to calculate the norm based on your ideal weight to avoid overloading the kidneys. That is, if your actual weight is 100 kg (220 pounds) and your ideal weight is 80 kg (176 pounds), it's better to aim for 2.4 liters (81 US fl oz) of water per day. And it's even better to rely on your actual condition, lifestyle, and markers of dehydration (athletes should drink a bit more). One of the best indicators of the body's water balance is the color of

Invictus Equilibrium

urine. If it's light, there's enough water; if it's dark, dehydration is present. The difference is noticeable in the morning. After sleep, the body is almost always dehydrated and needs water, so drinking one or two glasses of water in the morning is very important.

Another marker of dehydration is dry skin. But you shouldn't flood yourself with water at the first signs of dehydration. Drink as much water as you want. It's important to understand that if you're used to drinking little water, you should increase your intake gradually. Drinking too much water is also not advisable. You can suffer from water intoxication, known as hyperhydration. There are cases of sudden deaths among athletes who drank very large amounts of water after competitions.

Some believe that different liquids like tea, juices, coffee, etc., should be counted as food rather than water, but I personally think differently, and studies confirm this. If a person consumes a sufficient amount of tea or coffee during the day and doesn't drink water at all, they do not show signs of dehydration. But it's important to remember that the best and most natural drink for our bodies is still water.

Oxidation-Reduction Potential

Oxidation-Reduction Potential (ORP) is the ability of a substance to oxidize or reduce another substance. For water, this is one of the indicators of contamination with impurities, but it's worth delving a bit deeper to truly understand the essence of all this.

At the electronic level, everything strives for stability. Substances that lack electrons seek to find them and are called free radicals or oxidants. Substances that have an excess of electrons seek to give them away and are called reducers or antioxidants.

A large number of free radicals in the body is not very beneficial. It can cause premature aging and lead to many diseases. That's why it's important to supply the body with a sufficient number of antioxidants to provide oxidants with the electrons they lack, thereby restoring normal chemical bonds between molecules.

ORP values less than zero indicate that the substance is a reducer (antioxidant), while values greater than zero indicate that the substance is an oxidizer (oxidant). The rate of oxidation or reduction of the body depends on the magnitude of the ORP value.

Invictus Equilibrium

The cells of our body have a negative oxidation-reduction potential. This value ranges from -150 to -300 mV (millivolts). Unfortunately, most tap water and even bottled water have a positive oxidation-reduction potential. And when water with a positive ORP enters our body, it begins to take free electrons from our body's cells, thereby destroying them. The more positive the ORP value of the water, the more harm oxidation brings to our body.

The ideal ORP values for water and food for our bodies are close to our internal ORP levels so that the body doesn't expend energy to reduce the potential of the water we drink but instead receives a charge of energy and benefit from it.

Examples of water with a negative ORP include meltwater and mountain spring water, which in most cases have a negative ORP. There are also many different bottles that, due to minerals, make the water's oxidation-reduction potential negative. Additionally, there are numerous filtration systems that can change the water's ORP. But it's important to understand that the best result cannot be achieved without actual ORP measurements using special devices.

pH

pH is a value that indicates the degree of acidity or alkalinity of a solution. A neutral solution is considered to have a pH of 7 units. All solutions with pH < 7 are acidic, and solutions with pH > 7 are alkaline. For example, the pH of our blood is approximately 7.4 units; stomach acid is 1.0–2.0; orange juice is 3.0; milk is 6.5–6.8; pure water is 7.0; bleach is 13.0.

The pH of the water you drink regularly should be in the range of 7.5 to 9.0 units. Water with a lower pH (distilled, boiled) lacks sufficient minerals necessary for our bodies. It's also harmful to consume mineral water with a higher pH on a regular basis, but if there are mineral deficiencies, periodic consumption can be beneficial. Such water is better consumed regularly only under a doctor's prescription. However, if the consumption of certain liquid is not constant, there's nothing wrong with liquids that have a higher or lower pH level. Maintaining the correct pH in the gastrointestinal tract prevents the development of various pathogenic organisms that feel uncomfortable in an alkaline environment. It's also worth noting that it's almost impossible to influence the pH of the blood, and a healthy body will always keep it within strict limits, regardless of the pH in all other parts of the body. The question is only about the resources the body spends on balancing acidity in one part or another.

The pH level can be measured using pH strips or electronic devices. I use a device that can measure both the pH and ORP of water.

Purification

Water should not be absolutely pure. The body must maintain a sodium-potassium balance. Through these and other salts, nerve impulses are conducted, and the water balance in our body's cells is maintained.

One option for obtaining good drinking water is to purify tap water and then mineralize and structure it. A good option for purification is a reverse osmosis membrane, but after it, we get water not only free of harmful microorganisms but also very purified water in which the amount of minerals and trace elements will be less than necessary for the normal functioning of our body.

Mineralization is simple. It's the process of saturating water with various minerals that must be present in water for the normal functioning of our body. There are many mineralizers available for sale, so everyone can find an option that suits them.

Regarding water structuring, this is about its "memory." Official science does not yet recognize this, and for me personally, it's also an incomprehensible process. On one hand, it's understandable, but on the other, it's not. But I certainly don't see how this process can harm you. In my opinion, there are only two options in such matters. Either it really works, and over time it will be scientifically confirmed, or you'll incur financial losses for a non-working device. And here it's actually just a matter of cost. If the price of a structurer is not high for you, you can say that you're not losing anything significant, and you might gain potential benefits. And we shouldn't forget about the placebo effect.

In conclusion to the entire chapter, I want to note that the best option is simple spring water, and our ancestors, in most cases, drank exactly that. Now it's a bit more complicated with spring water, but it's important to clearly understand that tea, coffee, sweet and carbonated water (even mineral water) are unnatural for us and, as a result, in most cases, harm our bodies in the long term. Therefore, the main drink in a healthy person's diet should be good plain non-carbonated water.

Chapter 9

Air

"The body can endure hunger and thirst, but without air - only a few minutes."

Hippocrates

Today, each of us has heard about the deterioration of air quality, and this is indeed a significant problem, especially in large cities. Poor air can reduce the expected lifespan by 2 to 7 years and can be the cause of many lung diseases that can substantially degrade your quality of life. Therefore, striving to breathe good, clean air is very important. It may not be obvious, but improving air quality is the simplest way to enhance overall health, productivity, and immunity.

It's also worth mentioning that you should always breathe through your nose. Nasal breathing oxygenates the brain, and as you already know, it controls your entire body.

So if you have nasal problems, you must address them. No matter how clean the air you breathe is, if you're not breathing through your nose, you'll never achieve maximum efficiency from your body. It should be noted that during high-intensity sports activities, it's normal to breathe through your mouth. The nose has limitations on the amount of air it can pass, and through the mouth, we can take in much more oxygen necessary for muscles under heavy loads.

Now let's examine more precisely what constitutes good, clean air. There are four main air quality indicators:

CO_2 Level: This indicates the amount of carbon dioxide in the air. Measured in ppm (parts per million).

tVOC: Total Volatile Organic Compounds. Natural gas, deodorant, paint fumes, formaldehyde emissions, and similar substances fall into this category. A standard household detector won't show the exact substance (there are many varieties), but if you spray deodorant near it or bring it close to an open gas burner, the readings will spike, serving as an indicator to identify the problem. Measured in mg/m^3.

PM2.5: This indicates microscopic solid particles about 2.5 micrometers in diameter (which is 20 times smaller than the diameter of a human hair). Simply put, it's super-fine dust in all possible forms. If you grind a stone in a blender, you'll get a lot of large dust and a lot of very small particles around 2.5 microns. Smoke from a bonfire also contains many unburned microscopic solid particles, which is clearly visible on a detector placed near the flame—the readings rise rapidly and significantly. Tiny pieces of asphalt, tire, and vehicle exhaust emissions also fall into this category.

Air Humidity: This is the amount of water vapor in the air. There is absolute humidity and relative humidity. Absolute humidity shows the exact amount of water vapor in a cubic meter, for example. Relative humidity shows the relative amount of moisture in the air as a percentage. Almost all household devices display relative humidity, so we'll only consider that.

CO_2

Monitoring the level of carbon dioxide in the air is quite important in today's world. In almost all indoor spaces, its level is significantly above normal. It's not lethal, but it greatly affects our body's functioning, especially productivity, stress tolerance, and, consequently, immunity.

If we look at the question of normal carbon dioxide levels from an evolutionary standpoint, we have very little actual data on the air our ancestors breathed. However, according to ice core studies, the CO_2 level during the period from 650,000 to 800,000 years ago was between 172–300 ppm, with an average value of about 250 ppm[1]. Whether this is low or high is hard to say, but the pre-industrial level (before 1750), which was about 280 ppm, is now considered the norm, and it's believed to have fluctuated around this number throughout human evolution, only sharply increasing after the 18th century. More active observations began in the 1960s, and the CO_2 level then was 315 ppm; now it's already 420 ppm.

The amount of carbon dioxide in clean forest air now is about 250–300 ppm. We can assume that our ancestors almost always breathed such air. The WHO standard for cities is around 400 ppm. They state a maximum acceptable level of 1,000–1,400 ppm. In reality, in most places where people are present (offices, schools, universities, stores), the actual CO_2 level exceeds 2,000 ppm, which affects us very negatively. There's a study showing that at CO_2 levels above 950 ppm, cognitive function indicators can drop by 15% compared to a level of 550 ppm, and at 1,400 ppm, the decline can reach 50%. And this refers to levels not exceeding 1,400 ppm[2]. At levels above 2,000 ppm, it's hard to talk about real productivity. If the brain slows down this much, we can assume that prolonged elevated CO_2 levels may impair the functioning of other parts of our body.

What conclusions should we draw? We should walk more often in the fresh air. Don't forget to ventilate the rooms you're in. In terms of numbers, aim to keep indoor CO_2 levels below 700–800 ppm, and ideally close to the outdoor level of 400–500 ppm.

PM2.5

This is essentially an indicator of mechanical air pollution. The problem with these particular particles is that they are so small that they can bypass our biological barriers and penetrate any organs of our body without hindrance. Our body accumulates them in the lungs and distributes them throughout the body. However, it's also worth noting that our body can cope with them if the exposure is not significant.

There are enough studies proving that purifying the air from mechanical particles leads to improved cognitive functions and reduces symptoms of already acquired lung diseases[3,4]. If the air in a room is heavily polluted, sleep quality drops significantly, making proper recovery very difficult[5,6].

Now a bit about the numbers. According to WHO standards, the annual average concentration for PM2.5 particles should not exceed 5 μg/m^3. Previously, the standard was 10 μg/m^3, which may suggest that even 5 μg/m^3 is not an ideal value. Therefore, I believe we should strive to purify the air in the rooms where we spend most of our time and try to avoid places where the air contains more than 5 µg/m³ of solid particles.

Practically speaking, it's better not to live permanently in large cities. Statistics show that in 92% of big cities, the air pollution index exceeds the norm. In practice, not everyone can leave cities, so it's definitely worth considering purchasing a household air purifier. In my personal opinion, buying this device is mandatory for most of the planet's population. No matter how clean the place you live is, air masses can travel thousands of kilometers. I personally have felt the sand from the Sahara on my teeth, even though it's at least 3,000 km away from me.

tVOC

The harm from volatile organic compounds is no less than from solid airborne particles. The most significant emissions of volatile compounds come from furniture (due to cheap varnishes and paints). To solve this problem, you can buy certified furniture that should contain fewer harmful substances, but in today's world, the chemical industry is developing very rapidly. New compounds are synthesized very quickly, and theoretically, it's quite possible to create a

Invictus Equilibrium

varnish containing compounds that simply won't be tested in a particular environmental certificate. That is, the certificate exists, but the emissions remain; it's just that the chemical formula has changed. Overall, I think certified furniture will still be slightly better than cheap analogs.

In practice, for most people, the most adequate method again is a household air filter that will purify what's already there and significantly reduce the impact of harmful compounds on the body.

There is no official standard for tVOC levels, but it's recommended to aim for values close to 0.5 mg/m^3. But as with everything, standards are good, but the lower the indicator, the better. However, this particular indicator without detailed analysis can give a false impression of air quality. Ordinary aromas from flowers during blooming can inflate the readings. Therefore, it's sensible to consider it and base judgments on the dynamics of the indicators.

Air Humidity

Breathing air with normal humidity is very important for our bodies. If you breathe overly dry air, it leads to the drying out of all mucous membranes, especially in the nose, and dries out your skin. Your skin and mucous membranes are the first line of immune defense. The simplest way to fight diseases is to prevent them from entering your body.

On the other hand, high humidity poses fewer threats to our bodies. Only with very high humidity does the body's thermoregulation worsen (sweat evaporates less effectively from the body). However, high indoor humidity leads to the active reproduction of various fungi, viruses, and bacteria, which can harm our bodies, and this should be paid attention to if you live in a very humid climate.

Wikipedia states that the optimal humidity for the human body is 40–60%, but this needs some clarification. This is the relative humidity indicator, and it's inaccurate. What's the essence of relative humidity? Air at different temperatures can hold different amounts of water vapor. For example, at a temperature of -10°C, one cubic meter of air can hold a maximum of 2.5 grams of water (at 100% humidity) in the form of vapor, while at +25°C, it can hold up to 23 grams of water.

Invictus Equilibrium

In fact, the most comfortable air for us has a humidity of 40–60% at a temperature of 18–25°C. In absolute terms, this means we need 6.5 grams to 14 grams of water per cubic meter of air. Why did I write all this? If you live in a country where the temperature never drops below +5°C throughout the year, then generally, humidity shouldn't concern you much. Just make sure you don't have mold in your house, and everything will be fine. But if, like me, you live in a country where -15°C is a normal temperature for a month, then you should pay attention to indoor humidity, especially during the cold season.

Outside, it's -10°C with 90% humidity. This means there's 2.25 grams of water in the air (2.5 grams * 90%). In your room, the temperature is 20°C, and when you ventilate it, you let in air with 2.25 grams of water vapor. The air heats up, but it doesn't contain more water; the relative humidity drops from 90% to less than 30%, which is very uncomfortable for the body both outdoors and indoors.

This issue can be resolved using a humidifier, but they're not without their issues. There are three main types of humidifiers: steam, ultrasonic, and evaporative (natural evaporation). I haven't found actual studies on the benefits or harms of specific types. But perhaps that's because humidifiers haven't been widely used for long, and there haven't been major scandals with them yet. In my opinion, evaporative humidifiers are the best option. Why? If we take steam humidifiers, they basically work like a kettle. The water heats up, evaporates, and humidifies the air. But any water (except distilled) will always contain various trace elements. When we drink them, if they're within normal limits, they benefit us. But when we heat water, these trace elements evaporate along with the water, and we then breathe them in. How different trace elements affect our bodies when we inhale too much of them is an open question.

Ultrasonic humidifiers work using an ultrasonic membrane, and during their operation, solid particles are released from the water into the air in even greater quantities than with steam humidifiers. All these data are not made up but have been experimentally verified. When an ultrasonic humidifier operates, the PM2.5 detector goes crazy. What consequences this might have for the body in the long term is unknown. My task is to convey information, and everyone can draw their own conclusions.

Chapter 10
The Body

"The body always tells the truth about how you treat it."

Louise Hay

Your body literally reflects your internal state and programs you. There's a study showing that if you stand for two minutes in an open pose (like champions at the Olympics), testosterone levels increase on average by 19%, and cortisol drops by 25%. Conversely, in closed poses, testosterone decreases by 10%, and cortisol increases by 17%[1]. Simply forcing a smile raises serotonin levels in the blood and lowers cortisol, reducing overall stress[2]. It's incredible, but the brain has a direct connection with the body. The body reflects the actual state of affairs in the brain, and through the body, you can program the brain. That's why the path to confidence should begin with posture.

In general, the body gives us many signals. Any deficiencies and changes in the body always manifest themselves. For example, dry skin on the hands may indicate insufficient air humidity or elevated sugar levels in the body or vitamin deficiencies. The causes are completely opposite, but the signal is the same. The essence of signals is not only to give you an exact answer but also to make you think about what has changed or what needs to change. With today's level of medicine and access to information, you can prevent a huge number of diseases before they cause significant harm to your body. Just listen to your body. Once is an accident, twice is a coincidence, three times is a pattern, four times is a law.

It's also worth mentioning one of the most common signals of our body. Everyone knows about it, but not everyone addresses it. And that is excess weight. It must be clearly understood that excess weight is not just a signal of overeating. It can result from poor sleep, hormonal imbalances, excessive stress, and that's certainly not the whole list. The point is that excess weight has an extremely strong impact on the body. Blood circulation in the brain decreases with increased body weight. In people with excess weight, the chances of developing many diseases increase. And if the amount of excess weight exceeds 30% of the norm, the risks multiply. It's important to be realistic. Completely eliminating the harmful effects of food, polluted air, stress, etc., on our body in today's world is extremely difficult, but these effects can be minimized. It's essential to understand that excess weight is not the only enemy of our health today, but its presence multiplies the potential harm from everything else.

Spinal Health

The spine is the foundation of our entire body. Taking care of your body should begin with addressing spinal problems. Central blood vessels, lymphatic channels, and major nerve endings run along the spine. Minor back problems can severely disrupt the functioning of internal organs. Each individual vertebra is connected to specific internal organs. You can look at numerous images online by searching "spine and organs," but it's important to understand that we are all different, and these images are not exact. However, they illustrate the point well. If you have liver problems, for example, the cause may simply be poor blood supply to the organ due to spinal issues.

Evolutionarily, our spine is designed for walking or running and is not adapted to prolonged sitting or lack of movement. For most people today, life is quite sedentary. It's also worth noting that very few of our ancestors lived to the age of 35+, and there's an assumption that our spine isn't very well adapted to a long life. However, if you monitor your spinal health, you can go a very long time without problems, and there are many living examples of people over 80 with quite healthy backs.

Spinal health is primarily about the muscular corset that supports it and relieving stress from existing critical points. It's not as important to have extremely strong back muscles as it is to avoid imbalances between the muscles of the front and back of the body. If you have strong chest muscles and very weak back muscles, you'll slouch because the chest muscles will pull your body forward. If you have a very weak abdomen, it won't be able to keep your body upright, and you'll also slouch. If you have poorly stretched muscles on the back of your thigh, your body will be pulled too far back, and this imbalance will be compensated by some part of your back. This is especially relevant for people with sedentary jobs, which are very common today. When you sit, the front part of your thigh is in an overstretched position, and the back part is contracted, which over time leads to actual changes in the sizes of muscles and ligaments, as our body is extremely adaptive and always adjusts as efficiently as possible to the conditions it is in. From this, we can conclude that short but regular stretching of your muscles and ligaments can solve many back problems. Personally, I stretch for 3 minutes 5 times a week, and this has actually eliminated all

Invictus Equilibrium

discomfort in my back. There are even studies showing that stretching one muscle group for more than 60 seconds doesn't make much sense[3]. When you stretch statically, somewhere after 35–45 seconds, the muscles seem to relax (you can feel this moment), and your brain receives a physical signal that a specific muscle needs to increase in size. About 5–10 seconds after that moment, you can finish stretching that muscle group. Also, don't forget that warmed-up muscles stretch better and are harder to injure, so it's good to stretch immediately after exercising or a brief warm-up.

There are many different imbalances, and to describe them all would require another book. But there are simple practices that very effectively stretch the spine, and if the problems aren't severe, they help over time to eliminate all discomfort. You just need to find your unique health routine.

From my experience, most of the best exercises for spinal health I've found in various yoga routines. Lately, I've settled on a set of exercises from Peter Kelder's book The Eye of Revelation (plus stretching the back of the thigh), and all my back discomfort has simply disappeared over time. It's a fairly simple set of exercises that very effectively stretch the spine and slightly train the muscular corset. It's also worth noting that I have a sports background and a fairly well-developed muscular corset, so I don't currently feel the need to add additional back or core exercises to this routine. You should realistically assess your own condition. Carefully examine your body. Monitor your posture and identify weak spots in the front of your body, the back, and in muscle flexibility. Don't focus too long on something if it doesn't bring results. We are all different, so only through trial and error can you find your formula.

There are also chairs with a single point of support. They're unstable, and your back is constantly engaged to maintain balance. I personally haven't used such solutions yet, but theoretically, they could work very well.

Sports and the Brain

Sports is a very important element of our lives because our bodies are evolutionarily designed for constant movement. If we compare our bodies with those of other primates, we are all perfectly adapted for marathon running. We have excellent muscular stabilization of the head, our spine is essentially a large spring, a small chest cavity to reduce air resistance, large gluteal muscles, long limbs, an excellent cooling system, and many other minor evolutionary adaptations. And if you ask the question, "Who is faster: a human or a horse?" most would say a horse. But in fact, over distances greater than 40 km, a trained human will almost always beat a trained horse. Over longer distances, horses

Invictus Equilibrium

simply have no chance; their bodies aren't adapted to such prolonged exertion. Even in Africa, there are still small numbers of tribes that hunt antelope simply by running them to exhaustion. They calmly catch up to the antelope; it starts to flee from them, but they continue running along its trail. They catch up again and force the antelope to flee, not allowing it to rest. After 15–20 km of continuous running, the antelope simply can't run any further due to fatigue and overheating. There's a hypothesis that such hunting was our evolutionary niche because our brain began to develop much later than our body.

There are numerous studies proving that even a single workout increases our intelligence. No one can clearly explain how exactly this happens, but it definitely does. Perhaps it's due to increased blood flow to the brain and, consequently, increased oxygen saturation. Or due to an increase in the speed of metabolic processes in the body, which can lead to an increase in neural connections. But the point is that physical activity boosts our intelligence levels. However, there's a nuance here. Studies on mice show that those who ran voluntarily developed their brains much better than those who were forced to[4]. So choose a sport you enjoy. There's also research involving runners who were asked to take a 10-day break from training. Even after just 10 days without exercise, their brain blood flow worsened, and as a result, cognitive abilities slightly declined[5]. Interestingly, the maximum increase in brain blood flow occurs at workloads ranging from 40% to 60% of maximum (there's a concept of maximum oxygen consumption (VO_2 max) by muscles; exact heart rate zones are determined individually in sports labs, but very roughly, the heart rate at VO_2 max can be calculated using the formula 220 minus your age). At workloads close to maximum (over 80% of VO_2 max), brain blood flow almost doesn't change (it initially increases, but when approaching peak loads, it decreases to the initial level). It's also worth noting that physical activity is beneficial for everyone, but for older people, exercise provides the most pronounced effect in improving brain function, while in children, the effect is barely noticeable. This may be because children naturally move a lot, and adding a little more doesn't significantly change anything.

So how much should you exercise? The absolute minimum is around 15 minutes a day. It's very detrimental for the brain if there's no increase in heart rate due to physical activity. The World Health Organization recommends 150 minutes of physical activity per week. Among the inhabitants of African hunter-gatherer tribes, which can still be found, there's approximately 133 minutes of physical activity per day. The truth lies somewhere in between, and it's different for everyone. For me, for example, it's about 400–500 minutes of physical activity per week. Twice a week, I play volleyball for fun (about 180 minutes total), and 2–3 times I walk from 6 km to 15 km. From what I know, brisk walking is the most beneficial exercise for our body (slow walking is also good, but the difference between brisk and slow walking is quite significant for the body), and I enjoy it, especially when walking in interesting places.

Sports and Immunity

While sports without overexertion is almost always beneficial for the brain, it's not so straightforward with immunity levels. In fact, after any physical exertion, our immunity decreases and takes 24–48 hours to recover, but it doesn't return to the previous level—it becomes slightly higher. So exercise acts as a stress factor for our immunity, and the body increases immunity levels in the future to counteract this. Long, exhausting workouts significantly suppress the immune system, and it takes longer to recover afterward. Here, the pattern is similar to that of blood flow in the brain. Workouts with moderate loads are the most effective.

Does this mean you should completely abandon, for example, strength training? Absolutely not. You just need to understand that after an exhausting workout, your chances of getting sick increase, and it's worth temporarily limiting contact with sick people or supporting your immunity with various supplements. Also, if you already have initial signs of illness (weakness, slight fever, etc.), physical exertion can worsen the situation. Seriously consider taking a 2–5 day break from training (it's very individual; just listen to yourself), or if you're a professional athlete, think about light training.

The World Health Organization divides people into children, adults, and very adults. Children (5–17 years old) are recommended to have at least 60 minutes of aerobic activity daily (running, brisk walking, cycling, swimming, jump rope). Adults (18–64 years old) are recommended 150–300 minutes of moderate-intensity aerobic activity per week or 75–150 minutes of high-intensity training, or a combination of both. For people 65+, 150 minutes of moderate intensity, 75 minutes of high intensity, or a mix.

In summary, the amount of training is a relative value. It's very important to understand that high-performance sports aren't associated with health; they're about something else entirely. For health, it's important not to push yourself into states of overtraining. If you feel you haven't recovered, don't be afraid to take a day off from exercise or reduce the load temporarily.

Hardening

Hardening is one of the few beneficial "drugs." Short-term exposure to cold or cold showers increases levels of dopamine and norepinephrine in the body as a protective reaction to stress, which can lead to positive changes in the body. Periodic exposure to cold in the long term boosts our immunity, reduces stress levels, can help with weight loss, increases testosterone, improves insulin sensitivity, and has many other effects that positively impact our health[6,7,8]. Here, the story is similar to exercise. Initially, there's a short-term decrease in immunity, followed by an increase with a margin. First, a short-term increase in stress levels, then a decrease.

From an evolutionary standpoint, the effect of cold on our body isn't very obvious. Our ancestors mostly lived in warm climates. Physically, cold should slow down all processes in our body, but in fact, the opposite happens. When we start to get cold, our body receives a signal that we're physically approaching thermal death and begins to mobilize resources. It's important to understand that cold exposure shouldn't be constant. Prolonged stress breaks down the body. Even after 45 seconds of cold exposure, clear positive changes are observed, which are almost indistinguishable from longer exposure (although some studies state that the best effects are observed in the 3–10 minute range). Even a few times a week is sufficient. Cold truly increases motivation and a natural lust for life. Conversely, everyone knows that working under high temperatures is very difficult.

Personally, I currently only practice contrast showers. I start with hot water and finish with cold (about 60–90 seconds). It wakes me up better than coffee and gives a lot of energy. It's important to understand that this is still stress, and you shouldn't engage in cold exposure practices 4–6 hours before sleep. Also, during the active phase of illnesses, it's worth taking a break. Don't overload your body.

Contraindications to cold exposure include cardiovascular problems. After exposure to cold, blood vessels initially constrict and then dilate. Therefore, if your blood vessels aren't in good condition due to alcohol, nicotine, or other reasons, you should be very cautious with cold exposure. After sudden cold exposure, blood circulation changes in the body, and if you have hidden problems with blood supply to internal organs, they may manifest after starting cold exposure practices. I don't think you need to be overly afraid of this; just monitor your body's signals. In fact, cold exposure can reveal your weak spots at early stages. Gradually increase the level of cold exposure to your body, avoid hypothermia, monitor reactions, and you'll be fine.

Invictus Equilibrium

Everything is individual. Just find the duration and water temperature that suit you.

Sweat

The largest organ for eliminating metabolic waste from our body is the skin. Therefore, it's very important to sweat periodically. Through sweat, our body removes many harmful substances and regulates heat exchange. Exercise should be intense enough to cause sweating. You can also periodically visit a sauna. Within reasonable limits, it can be beneficial.

Normally, our sweat doesn't have a very strong odor and doesn't cause great aversion. If your sweat has a sharp and specific smell, it's often a signal that something isn't working properly in the body. If the glands can't cope with eliminating toxins, they may be excreted through sweat, worsening the smell. A bad odor can also indicate poor diet or insufficient water intake. It's important to understand that sweat also washes out useful trace elements, so if your workouts are high-intensity and last more than 60 minutes, it makes sense to periodically add electrolytes to your diet to restore their balance.

It's also necessary to mention antiperspirants and deodorants. Deodorants simply mask odors and essentially don't interfere with the body's functions, so they can be considered safe (until proven otherwise). With antiperspirants, it's a bit more complicated. They actually affect the work of sweat glands and, as a result, reduce sweating. This happens mainly due to aluminum salts that block sweat glands. They're considered safe, but research continues. In fact, there are quite a few studies suggesting they can affect our endocrine glands and may provoke the development of breast cancer. All studies are quite questionable, but their very existence should make you think. User reviews also indicate that many people experience skin problems after use, directly indicating that not everything is entirely safe since antiperspirants physically interfere with gland functions. And as has happened many times: "What is considered safe today may not necessarily remain so tomorrow."

Personally, I don't use any. Evolutionarily, sweat wasn't masked in any way. It should come out. Sweat itself has no odor. The smell is formed due to the activity of microorganisms (referring to the skin microbiome, more on this later) that live on human skin, serve as the first immune barrier, and essentially feed on sweat. That's why using antibacterial soap doesn't always bring benefits because it aggressively fights not only harmful bacteria but also beneficial ones, which can lead to various skin problems due to the disruption of the natural barrier. It's also worth mentioning that sweat is a natural aphrodisiac. Therefore, I believe it's necessary to monitor not the sweat that comes out but the body from which it comes.

Bioimpedance Analysis

Bioimpedance analysis is a method for rapid assessment of human body composition. It works by measuring electrical resistance between different parts of the body. Using this method, you can measure the amount of fat, fluid, muscle tissue, metabolic rate, and bone mass in the body. The device that performs these measurements is called a bioimpedance meter.

From a practical standpoint, these measurements can be an interesting addition for tracking your progress during various body transformations. In moments when, for example, weight loss has stalled, such measurements can help you understand whether the balance of muscle and fat tissue in the body is changing. It often happens that body volumes decrease, but weight doesn't because muscles are simply heavier than fat.

There are many devices for bioimpedance measurement on the market, but it's important to understand that none of them provide exact results. Deviations can reach up to 9%. If you measure a person on an empty stomach, then drink 1 liter (33 fl oz) of water and measure again, the results will differ. But if you use this device as a marker of changes, taking measurements under the same conditions, these data can be quite useful overall. It can really simplify the process of tracking the effectiveness of certain methods specifically for your body.

Clothing

There's an interesting proven effect of transference of feelings. This is when you start to feel certain emotions when interacting with a specific object. Cake is associated with celebration; fireworks - with New Year or weddings. There's a very popular study that showed that associating oneself with a certain big brand can temporarily increase cognitive abilities[9]. Different groups were shown logos of famous brands and then given tests. There was a brand that reliably increased the cognitive abilities of the group that was shown it before taking the test.

If we approach this effect from an evolutionary standpoint, an individual personality in nature simply doesn't exist. Our ancestors always lived in communities (tribes), and this is very logical. Surviving alone in the wild and passing on genes through generations is simply impossible. Everyone

Invictus Equilibrium

in the community associated themselves with it. Joy was shared, and sorrow was shared. This is also confirmed. There's a study that reliably shows that after a football match, men who supported the winning team experience an increase in testosterone levels. Those who supported the losing team see a decrease in testosterone[10]. Therefore, after this, I personally only root for the winners.)

It's a similar story with clothing. Society has penetrated us so deeply that we'll always perceive a person in a business suit a bit more seriously. But in fact, the essence is slightly different. Clothing gives us the power we attribute to it or that our environment attributes to it. There are studies where schools introduced uniforms and changed nothing else. As a result, students' academic performance improved[11,12]. You could say that the school uniform has a magical effect, but I think these results should be interpreted differently. Our brain works much better if we separate environments, and it also very effectively connects seemingly unrelated things. If a student always studies in the same uniform and does nothing else in it, the brain begins to clearly associate that clothing with the learning process. As a result, after the student puts on the uniform, the brain starts to concentrate on performing a specific task, leading to increased efficiency in the learning process because there's constant reinforcement of the image through action. It turns out that if you consistently exercise in certain attire, your brain will more effectively prepare your body for training. If you try to work in clothes in which you always relax, your work efficiency may decrease. It's easier for the brain to work when you emphasize different processes with different objects and images. Therefore, if you have items associated with stress or unpleasant events, it's worth getting rid of them.

Regarding the physical impact of clothing on the body, I don't know much data, but there are quite accurate findings that tight underwear in men leads to decreased sperm quality and testosterone levels[13], and in women, it can lead to various diseases due to impaired blood circulation and changes in microclimate. It's important to understand that anything that changes the natural position of our body can alter our internal state through hormonal balance.

Clothing has the power you give it. If you're psychologically ready to succeed in society, it doesn't matter what clothes you're wearing. Don't let fashion shape you. Shape fashion!

Sex

Sex is another free and harmless "drug" for our body. It lifts mood, reduces cortisol levels, improves sleep, and much more. Sex combined with love for a partner has an even

Invictus Equilibrium

greater effect and significantly impacts the quality of our life as a whole. Let's not delve into details. The process, in its basic form, isn't very complicated. Sex reflects our basic evolutionary need for reproduction, and our psychological state is very closely tied to it. It should definitely be part of everyone's life, and masturbation doesn't replace it. It's worth writing a bit about that.

There are many opinions and studies showing that masturbation is harmful or beneficial, and I don't aim to argue strongly with them; I just want to convey my perspective on this process. Our body and brain are inseparably connected. Although during sex our body releases significantly more hormones than during masturbation, for our brain, these are very similar processes. It turns out that when you masturbate instead of having sex, you're sending a signal to your brain that everything is fine in your life and your struggle for sexual selection is temporarily over. I don't know exactly how it is for girls, but for guys, during abstinence (we're talking about periods not exceeding a few months), testosterone levels often increase, which may indicate natural mechanisms to increase the likelihood of success in sexual selection. But you need to be careful with all this. If you don't sublimate (redirect) the increased amount of energy you receive as a result of abstinence, you might get the opposite effect. We're all different, and in such matters, you need to closely monitor what signals you're sending to your brain through your body and what reactions you receive. The brain gave you energy through increased testosterone, and you didn't use it. What feedback did your brain receive?

The reproductive function is one of the basic ones in our body, and the brain can often focus on it. If you can't reproduce, then all other processes aren't as important, thinks our brain. Therefore, if you have a healthy reproductive system, this will be a very good signal for your brain. It will do everything possible to help you adjust all other processes because, in its understanding, your main biological mission isn't yet complete. To keep your reproductive system in good condition for a long time, don't forget about the tone of your pelvic floor muscles, as a sedentary lifestyle doesn't contribute to their development. Kegel exercises are a good option.

It's also worth mentioning pornography. It's definitely harmful. Addiction can definitely form from watching it[14]. Importantly, it has an extremely strong impact on your internal state, motivation level, and actually changes your brain. When you watch porn, your brain essentially receives a signal that there are plenty of females or males in your life. Your brain doesn't distinguish reality from the image, and after receiving the illusion that you've won sexual selection,

Invictus Equilibrium

it can significantly, through changes in your hormonal balance, affect your level of motivation and, more importantly, your zest for life. Regarding the formation of dopamine addiction, I won't even start. There's a wonderful saying, "A poet must be hungry," which well reflects the essence of many evolutionary adaptations of our species. But overall, sex is good. Have sex, but not alone.

Chapter 11
Nutrition

"We are what we eat."
Hippocrates

Nutrition is one of the very important pieces in forming a healthy body. In fact, eating right isn't difficult. The problem for most of us in today's world is that we've been taught to eat improperly, and we've gotten used to it. Pizza, burgers, soda, and similar foods bring great harm to our bodies. For example, when it comes to immunity, our intestines contain Paneth cells, which play a very important role in providing antibacterial protection. They secrete antimicrobial substances and help maintain the intestinal barrier. Studies show that a Western diet (high in fat, sugar, and fast carbohydrates) disables the functions of Paneth cells, which significantly reduces immune responses[1]. However, most of us are so accustomed to all this that we're not ready to rethink the essence of our nutrition in one day and switch to healthy foods. But recognizing the problem is the first step to solving it. Let's get to it.

Invictus Equilibrium

First, it's important to understand that food shouldn't be the essence of our lives. It can enhance our lives but shouldn't come first. In my opinion, food should be perceived simply as energy; otherwise, we become slaves to our stomachs. But we shouldn't disrespect it either, because it's thanks to food that we live.

On one hand, I don't think we need to completely give up tasty food (although healthy food can also be very tasty). Just don't make it a daily routine. No matter how you look at it, delicious food causes large releases of dopamine in our brains and, as a result, can lead to addiction. So it's like a mild drug, and we should be careful with it. Consuming such "drugs" every day certainly won't be beneficial, but if you do it once a month or a few times, there won't be noticeable harm, and the pleasure will be many times greater.

But on the other hand, we should completely try to move away from such thoughts. This logic is somewhat flawed. If you fill up a car with poor-quality fuel just once, it will always leave its consequences; they may not manifest immediately (carbon deposits begin to form on the spark plugs, etc.—car enthusiasts will understand the analogy). A burger once a week will still cause harm. It's impossible to glue a chipped cup so that the chip isn't visible. Our body isn't a cup or a car; it's a bit more complex, but the point I want to convey is that everything has its resource, and it's not infinite.

And, in my opinion, the question is only what you exchange your resource for. Nature is ruthless (but I believe it's fair), and whatever you do, it will make you exchange your personal resource. The question is at what exchange rate. Is that piece of cake worth the emotions you'll get from it? If you don't understand why you need to live to 100 years or why you should increase your chances of celebrating New Year on Mars, for example, that's your right. You just need to ask yourself honest questions. How long do you plan to live? How? Why? And what are you doing today to achieve that?

It's also worth saying that no matter how morally strong you are, you should also understand that our stomach can control us. This is not just words. It actually affects your decisions. There's an interesting study that vividly shows this. Researchers studied judges' decisions when considering parole cases. More than 1,100 decisions were reviewed, and a very clear pattern was found. Prisoners whose cases were heard first thing in the morning had about a 65% chance of a positive decision, while those whose cases were heard right before lunch had chances close to zero. And cases considered immediately after lunch again had about a 65% chance of a positive result, and then the probability decreased with a clear correlation to the judge's satiety. In other words, the freedom of certain prisoners completely depended on whether the judge was hungry or full[2]. And it can be confidently said that the stomach affects not only judges' decisions but yours as well. So don't forget to feed the person from whom you plan to borrow something.

I am also convinced that there is no basic type of nutrition that would suit everyone. We are all different; we have different stomach acidities, different metabolic rates, etc. But there are definitely things that don't suit any of us and that, unfortunately, are deeply rooted in our society and gradually kill us. Therefore, we'll further figure out what suits everyone and what doesn't. And you'll assemble the final puzzle yourself.

Calories

A calorie is a unit of energy measurement. To determine the caloric content of products, they are simply burned, and the amount of energy released is calculated. After calculations, numbers indicating the caloric content in kilocalories are displayed on product packaging.

The World Health Organization recommends consuming 1,700–2,000 kcal per day for women, 2,500–2,600 kcal per day for men, and 1,500–2,000 kcal for children. In fact, these values are conditional and should serve as a guideline. It's more important to focus on maintaining a balance between energy expended and energy received, and on the actual state of your body. It is the best marker. If you consume more than the norm but don't have excess weight and you need an increased number of calories (you're an athlete or do hard physical work), this can be justified.

There are many opinions and studies regarding how many times a day one should eat. In fact, frequent meals (4–6 times) in small portions can be quite beneficial. This works especially well for disorders of the gastrointestinal tract, diabetes, as dietary nutrition, etc. But overall, I believe that 2–3 meals a day are normal for most people. If you look at this issue from an evolutionary standpoint, I'm sure our ancestors didn't have long periods of constant satiety. Therefore, I lean toward the idea that short periods of hunger are normal and even necessary for our bodies. It's also important to consider that it's better to eat at approximately the same time so that the body is better prepared.

It's also worth adding that you shouldn't consume very hot drinks and food in general. For most people, anything above 65°C will be considered hot. Hot food injures the mucous membranes, which can lead to a large number of diseases related to the gastrointestinal tract, including various types of cancer. It's better for everything that enters your body to be just warm.

The question of distributing calories throughout the day is also essentially individual, but as practice shows, most people do better when they consume the fewest calories in the morning and the most in the evening. Some even completely skip breakfast and have a lot of energy throughout the day, and only in the second half of the day begin to replenish their reserves. Personally, I also feel much better with a light breakfast.

Fats, Proteins, and Carbohydrates

It's very important to maintain balance in nutrition and provide the body with all macronutrients (which are essentially fats, proteins, and carbohydrates). The daily norm is considered to be 1–1.5 grams of protein per 1 kg of body weight, 0.8–1.5 grams of fats per 1 kg of body weight, and 2 grams of carbohydrates per 1 kg of body weight. In fact, all recommendations regarding the amount of proteins, fats, carbohydrates, and calories are conditional. They heavily depend on lifestyle. And if we convert proteins, fats, and carbohydrates into calories, the recommendations often don't match. The calculation is simple: 1 gram of protein equals 4.1 kcal, 1 gram of carbohydrates equals 4.2 kcal, 1 gram of fat equals 9.3 kcal. For example, for my 70 kg: 1.5*70*4.1 = 430 kcal from proteins, 2*70*4.2 = 588 kcal from carbohydrates, and 1.5*70*9.3 = 976 kcal from fats. As a result, 1,994 kcal, which is already insufficient compared to the norm of 2,500 kcal, and if you add sports, you get a normal deficit. But in reality, this may be enough for someone, and that's why I recommend focusing more not on calories but on the actual state of your body, how you feel, and focusing more on the usefulness of the macronutrients consumed and their balance. It's recommended that the diet consists of 30% proteins, 30% fats, and 40% carbohydrates. This is closer to reality because if, for example, you had a hard day today, you need more energy; if it's a day off, you need less. But still, the main thing will be the quality of the macronutrients, and here it's worth delving into more detail.

For example, carbohydrates are divided into two types: simple and complex. Simply put, complex carbohydrates have a more complex structure and can't be quickly absorbed, so they are first broken down into simpler compounds, and because of this, they don't cause large spikes in insulin and glucose in the blood. These include various grains, mushrooms, legumes, whole-grain bread, nuts, brown rice, and similar foods. With simple carbohydrates, it's the opposite. These are compounds that break down very quickly and lead to a rapid increase in glucose and insulin levels in our blood. These include all products with a high sugar content, soda, pastries, etc. It's better to consume complex carbohydrates and minimize the amount of simple ones.

We are essentially protein structures, so the presence of protein in our diet is very important. All proteins consist of amino acids, which are divided into essential and non-essential. The main thing to note here is that there are plant

Invictus Equilibrium

and animal proteins. Some amino acids necessary for our body are only found in animal protein. They cannot be replaced by plant protein. In fact, plant protein is incomplete, so the presence of at least a small amount of animal protein in a healthy person's diet is mandatory for normal body functioning.

Regarding fats, they are divided into three main groups: saturated, unsaturated, and trans fats. Trans fats are mostly unhealthy. They are mainly fats that have been processed from regular fats. They are found in cookies, mayonnaise, refined vegetable oil, chocolate, margarine, butter, and similar products. Their consumption should be avoided. On the other hand, saturated and unsaturated fats are beneficial and necessary in certain amounts for our bodies. Saturated fats are present in eggs, meat, dairy products, etc. Unsaturated fats include Omega-3, Omega-6, and Omega-9. They are found in nuts, avocados, fish, olives, seeds, etc. Unsaturated fats are considered the most beneficial.

It's also worth mentioning cholesterol. Most people equate cholesterol with fat, but in fact, it's a completely different compound that is necessary in certain amounts for our bodies. Cholesterol is used to synthesize a large number of different hormones, form cell membranes, contribute to the synthesis of vitamin D, and much more. In general, cholesterol is one of the types of natural alcohols and is easily synthesized by our bodies from fats, amino acids, or glucose. 80% of cholesterol is synthesized in our liver, and the rest we get from food. But it's important that the level of cholesterol, like everything else, isn't too low or too high. Good sources of cholesterol include eggs, cod liver oil, fatty fish, and other animal products. But to prevent high cholesterol levels, it's worth having a lot of fiber in your diet (these are all vegetables and fruits). The World Health Organization recommends at least 400 grams of vegetables and fruits per day. There is also an opinion that elevated cholesterol indicates the presence of some other inflammatory process in the body that it is trying to solve by increasing cholesterol levels.

When it comes to distributing macronutrients throughout the day, it's individual, but for most people, it's better to consume the majority of their daily carbohydrate intake at breakfast. These should be complex carbohydrates. And shift the consumption of most proteins and fats to the second half of the day, with more at dinner. About 70% of the daily protein norm should be animal proteins (eggs, dairy products, meat, etc.), and the rest plant-based. With fats, it's the opposite. Approximately 35% of fats from the daily norm should be animal fats (fish, meat, dairy products, etc.), and the rest plant-based fats.

If we approach the issue of nutrition from an evolutionary standpoint, the most beneficial food for us is the

Invictus Equilibrium

simplest products. The less processed the food, the better for our bodies. The body should spend more energy on unprocessed food, which helps it maintain the correct microflora in the intestines, which significantly affects our immunity. Unprocessed food also contains more vitamins and minerals. Our ancestors didn't have salt (its consumption actually needs to be limited[3]), spices, flavorings, preservatives, thickeners, and similar additives. They ate simply roasted meat or fish, many raw vegetables and fruits. And only relatively recently, if we consider the entire period of our evolution, did they learn to cook various porridges and bake bread. And those cooking methods differed greatly from today's. Bread was always made from very coarsely ground flour, which can be beneficial compared to refined flour. And porridges were often simply steamed, which essentially preserved a larger number of beneficial substances. But the main diet was still based on hunting and gathering.

Microbiome

The microbiome is a community of microorganisms that live together in a particular habitat. Synonyms are microflora, microbiota. Each of us has unique microbiomes in our stomachs, on our skin, in our nasopharynx. And this is actually a very important topic. Extremely important. Because your stomach controls you. And that's the truth!

According to recent estimates, about 40 trillion different bacteria live in our bodies, while there are 30 trillion cells in our bodies. Just try to imagine that number. More microorganisms live on and inside your body than the cells of your entire body. And this number doesn't yet account for various viruses and fungi that are potentially also present in our bodies. Isn't this another organ, at least? If not another organism that simply lives in symbiosis with us.

In our stomach alone, there are about 2 kg of various bacteria, and they constantly synthesize some substances (they can digest complex carbohydrates, synthesize fatty acids, vitamins, and even toxic substances) that, in one way or another, affect our bodies. If the body is deprived of its microbiome, a person will die within a few hours. That's why the microbiome is sometimes called a separate organ. And it's very important to understand whom you're feeding there or whom you're killing if we're talking about alcohol, for example. Alcohol actually greatly changes the microbiome. Studies show that the number of beneficial bacteria decreases significantly after alcohol consumption, while the number of pathogenic ones increases[4]. There's also research showing that altered microbiota after alcohol consumption increases voluntary alcohol consumption in the future, which essentially indicates the formation of alcohol dependence at the microbiome level[5]. This indirectly proves that the microbiome can influence our thoughts, desires, and actions by changing the chemical composition of our blood, supplying various substances there regardless of whether we like it or not. And essentially, if you don't understand this, riding this horse will not be easy.

For example, there's the parasite Toxoplasma, which is mostly spread through felines and can cause the disease toxoplasmosis. It usually occurs in a rather mild form, but sometimes lethal outcomes are possible. There's a study proving that the presence of this parasite in the body can lead to changes in the host's appearance and behavior. It talks about improved facial symmetry in men and a decrease in the average body mass index in women. Tests also show that infected men and women are rated as more attractive. And since this parasite is transmitted sexually, this increases its chances of spreading[6].

The structure of the microbiome affects our psyche and even our behavior. Bacteria in our stomach can actually control us by influencing our mood until we eat certain foods that will promote their survival (mostly, this will be unhealthy food)[7]. There's a study proving that after taking antibiotics, people may experience depression and increased anxiety, which is directly related to the fact that antibiotics kill the microflora of our stomach[8]. Experiments on rats also confirm this effect, at least in those prone to anxiety. After antibiotic therapy, negative changes occurred in the animals' immune systems and behavior (mainly increased anxious behavior)[9]. All this sounds atypical, but the microbiota in your stomach can actually significantly affect processes in your brain. And this influence occurs from your birth to your death[10]. And there's no single standard here (at least not yet). You need to create your unique microbiota that will meet your needs. And its formation will greatly depend on your eating habits, the amount of physical activity, sleep, and other physical needs of your body. Simply by understanding how it all works, you can greatly increase the effectiveness of your actions with the help of supplements, gradual rejection of harmful things, and similar measures. And with a higher probability, you can achieve the desired life result.

You also need to understand that "correct" microorganisms can't properly digest conditional fast food;

Invictus Equilibrium

this is well illustrated by the "Happy Meal" experiment. In it, an American woman bought fast food and stored it. After 6 years, when she opened the box, she saw that the food had hardly spoiled, and the packaging began to decompose before the food. If we take food and simply leave it in the open air, and ordinary microorganisms don't eat it (as evidenced by the fact that it doesn't spoil), then what kind of microorganisms should be in our stomach to digest it when we eat it? For "correct" microorganisms, this is an impossible task. But pathogens, as research shows, quickly adapt to different environments, and essentially, normal microflora is replaced by pathogenic flora. And then, forming normal microbiota after switching to proper nutrition takes quite a long time.

At first, the benefits of proper nutrition may be minimal because there aren't enough microorganisms that can properly digest beneficial substances. And on the other hand, when you have formed a large number of pathogenic microorganisms that, for example, love sugar, during the period when you give it up, they may even release toxic substances into the blood, which can cause headaches, weakness, and other effects that can be conditionally compared to drug withdrawal. Returning to a normal microbiota can take even as long as it took you to grow the pathogenic one. This can actually be a long time. But the first significant changes in microflora can occur within 4–6 weeks. This is the minimum term for changes.

Now, the method of microbiota transplantation through feces is also gaining popularity, but it's under-researched and has certain nuances. From what I've seen, there are studies with positive results and some with not so positive ones. Personally, I believe that the issues of the microbiome are very complex overall, and such radical methods, until there is very clear evidence of their effectiveness or critical necessity, I definitely wouldn't use. And I also believe that the natural way of changing the microbiome is safer and more correct. Even when you specifically try to introduce certain bacteria from supplements into your microflora, you don't disrupt the natural course of things and the natural competition within your body. It's like eating some specific fruit or vegetable and slightly changing the balance of microflora in your stomach. And whether those bacteria will take root is already a question of how you will feed and protect them so that they can win the competitive struggle in your microbiome and bring you the desired benefit.

Our body and immune system as a whole are extremely complex systems that we don't fully understand yet. At first glance, it may seem that there shouldn't be pathogenic bacteria and parasites in our microbiome, but in fact, this can

Invictus Equilibrium

cause serious disruptions in the immune system. Parasites in the body play an extremely important role in forming the immune response. Essentially, it's like a gym for our immune system. It should always be in good shape, but at the same time, it's necessary to control the load that parasites create inside you. And again, we come to balance. And it will greatly depend on which microorganisms you feed in your body. Which group will dominate? If your life includes sports, good sleep, good nutrition, little stress, and overall a good psycho-emotional balance, then essentially, all attempts to eliminate conditional parasites from your body may bring more harm than good.

Don't forget that frequent exposure to various chemicals in our bodies can lead to resistance to them. In simple terms, you're not only killing your parasites but also training them to resist. An adequate option for parasite prevention without a specific medical diagnosis can be the use of various natural bitter herbs and vegetables like garlic, onions, or pumpkin seeds. In different regions of the planet, there are different options, and if you have a great desire or, in your opinion, a need to fight parasites, this would be a good option if done without fanaticism. This method is more about suppressing them to optimal levels for your body rather than total elimination. Therefore, 1–2 similar therapies a year, if you feel the need, are unlikely to bring more harm than good.

Probiotics and Prebiotics

As you may have already understood, bacteria play an extremely important role in our lives. They significantly affect our immunity, metabolism, and even intellect and mood. Therefore, it makes sense to figure out how you can influence your own microflora. To do this, you need to understand what probiotics and prebiotics are.

Probiotics are live microorganisms that, when consumed in sufficient quantities, can benefit the host's health. They maintain the balance of beneficial bacteria in the intestines and help fight various pathogens. Probiotics also improve digestion, synthesize certain vitamins, protect against pathogens, support immunity, and much more. Probiotics include bifidobacteria (maintain stomach acidity, which hinders the growth of harmful bacteria), lactobacilli (participate in the synthesis of B-group vitamins and stimulate the immune system), saccharomycetes (help restore microflora, for example, after taking antibiotics), streptococci (help digest dairy products), and many others.

Prebiotics are indigestible food components (mainly various fibers) that probiotics feed on, which helps beneficial bacteria reproduce better and function more effectively. Consuming prebiotics can lead to improved metabolism, increased immunity, and better digestion. The main sources

Invictus Equilibrium

of prebiotics are various grains, vegetables, fruits, nuts, and seeds.

It's also worth noting that probiotics and prebiotics can be in the form of supplements, and their use can be quite effective. They can be taken separately or as synbiotics, which are essentially a combination of probiotics and prebiotics to increase effectiveness. This is actually an effective way to speed up changes in your microflora. For example, not so long ago, scientists discovered a specific strain of Streptococcus salivarius (BLIS K12) in the mouths of healthy people. Studies have shown that it effectively supports ear, throat, and nose health, helps maintain fresh breath, and improves local immunity[11].

Regarding the safety of probiotics from supplements in general, in my personal conviction, their intake is quite safe. Although I haven't found studies that I consider adequate regarding the safety of probiotics, I also haven't found any normal studies about their danger. In the studies I have seen, the formulations are very similar and cautious. They write that no obvious negative effects have been identified, although isolated cases of individual intolerance occur. Therefore, I personally concluded for myself that such things can be used when needed, just monitoring possible reactions of your body more closely.

Sugar

No matter how much we all (or not all) love sweets, unfortunately, they kill our bodies and steal our energy, even though it seems the opposite. Evolutionarily, our brain is set up to reward us for consuming high-calorie food, and any food with a lot of calories causes dopamine releases in us and brings pleasure. Previously, this was an evolutionary necessity, but now, when most people on the planet don't have a calorie deficit, it makes us weak and unhappy.

Most of the problems from high-calorie food are brought to us by sugar and fast carbohydrates (sugar is essentially fast carbohydrates). In nature, there is no refined sugar or products with high sugar concentrations, so our body is absolutely unadapted to large amounts of it. When you simply eat something tasty, you get a small dose of dopamine, but when you consume a sugar-containing product, due to the large number of calories that are immediately broken down, you get a huge spike in dopamine, and then a very big drop. All this contributes to the formation of addiction and can cause various depressive states, which is scientifically proven. There are studies according to which sugar addiction is greater than cocaine addiction. Sugar is a drug![12,13]

Sugar not only breaks the nervous system but also greatly worsens the state of our bodies. Fast carbohydrates accelerate the processes of collagen destruction and, as a result, worsen the quality of skin and hair. Sugar accelerates inflammatory processes and worsens wound healing. Sugar is an ideal environment for the development of any microorganisms. But as studies show, bad microorganisms develop at a much higher rate than good ones thanks to it[14]. If giving up sweets is very difficult and there's a constant desire to consume them, this is one of the symptoms of the presence of parasites in the body that manipulate you. Sugar, in the long term, destroys our brain, despite the fact that in the short term it can give us instant energy. And these are definitely not all the negative consequences of consuming sugar.

It's actually not easy for any of us to give up sweets. The only natural product that is both fatty and sweet is mother's milk, and our brain remembers this well. That's why it's very hard for us psychologically to resist fatty and sweet foods. And it turns out that the most adequate way to fight this is the absence of harmful forms of it in your home. You need to be as radical as possible. If there's a gun hanging on the wall, it will eventually fire. Everything in your home will be eaten by someone sooner or later, at least until you completely rethink mentally and physically your eating habits.

Also, don't forget to look at product compositions. Today, a very large number of products have huge amounts of sugar. Its amount is easy to calculate. Look at the amount of carbohydrates, and in fact, you see the amount of sugar. If you look at the label, for example, of a well-known red soda and see the number 10.3 grams of carbohydrates per 100 grams of product, know that this is 10.3 grams of pure sugar. And if you look at the labels of products in your refrigerator, you'll be surprised how much sugar is, for example, in ordinary ketchup. This simple formula works with almost all products that definitely don't have complex carbohydrates in their composition. Carbohydrates in porridge will be different.

Considering all that's written, it's safe to say that giving up sugar-containing products will benefit everyone. Personally, I love sweets very much, and so far, I haven't been able to completely give them up. But I have a few rules that greatly reduce dependence and consumption of sugar-containing products. I don't have sweets in my house. If I want something sweet, I must walk to the store at least 1 km (plus the same distance back), and then I can buy conditional ice cream. But the ideal option for me is consuming sweets only on holidays a few times a year. A piece of cake on your birthday is incredibly tasty if you haven't eaten sweets for more than a month before that. And you get pleasure, there's no desire to eat a lot of sweets, and the long-term harm is very small.

Invictus Equilibrium

Regarding tests, a blood sugar level above 7 mmol/L is already considered to indicate type 2 diabetes. The norm is considered to be 3.9–5.5 mmol/L after 8–10 hours of fasting. In my opinion, anything above 5–5.2 mmol/L should signal you to think about whether everything is okay with your diet. These are not yet critical levels, but already a signal to start monitoring its level and gradually adjust your diet and lifestyle if your goal is to be healthy, of course. You also need to understand that consuming refined sugars increases deficiencies of zinc, magnesium, chromium because they are necessary for sugar processing in the body, and their deficiencies can lead to related problems that will actually be associated with sugar consumption.

When it comes to sugar substitutes, I consider natural stevia to be the best option. Some people talk about brown cane sugar as a substitute for regular sugar, but in fact, this doesn't change anything. Their caloric content is almost identical. If we mention all other chemical sugar substitutes and sweeteners (there are actually many of them), there are many studies that talk about their safety. Conversely, there are enough studies that prove their harm. If we approach this issue from a logical standpoint, chemical sweeteners are cheaper than sugar, and they are more profitable for product manufacturers. There is very little data on who sponsors certain studies, and it's unknown whether there's any financial interest involved. In fact, when you consume a sugar substitute, you're deceiving your brain. It thinks you've received many calories, but in fact, there's nothing in the stomach. And as a result, you can get many disorders associated with addiction to sweets and disruptions in insulin hormone function. There are studies showing that insulin in the blood increases when sugar substitutes enter the body[15].

If we summarize, the issue of sugar substitutes is not fully researched. But considering the studies that already exist and the fact that these are unnatural compounds, I definitely wouldn't recommend consuming them on a regular basis. When I have a choice between sugar and a substitute, I always choose sugar. It's honest for our body, and I'm aware of its harm. The real harm from substitutes will be known more accurately only over time. The only adequate option for their use is temporarily replacing regular sugar with substitutes (if there are already contraindications to regular sugar) as one of the stages on the way to completely giving up sugar. Give up sugar and taste the real flavor of good food. Also, if this material hasn't convinced you or turned out to be quite complicated, there's a wonderful film "That Sugar Film" (2014), which convincingly highlights the harm of refined sugar but in a slightly different form.

Vegetarianism (and Similar Diets)

You need to eat plenty of vegetables and fruits—that's true. There are studies proving that the amount of fiber consumed significantly affects the overall level of happiness and health[16,17,18]. Plant-based food contains many vitamins and antioxidants that we need. However, as a large number of studies show, any types of diets lacking animal macronutrients are incomplete for our bodies and lead to various deficiencies. I don't aim to convince anyone of anything or describe the proven harm or benefits of diets without meat or with it. I just want to write about some logical contradictions I see in proponents of one-sided types of nutrition.

Plant protein is incomplete in its composition and cannot be compared to animal protein. Certain essential amino acids are present only in animal proteins and cannot be replaced (unless you consider supplements). Therefore, I personally believe that the presence of meat and fish in the diet is mandatory, but proponents of vegetarianism have many quite interesting and at first glance logical statements that explain our evolutionary unadaptedness to consuming meat.

There's a claim that our stomach isn't formed to digest raw meat, which means we don't need to consume it in any form. In fact, our stomach has one of the highest acidities among all known animals. Our stomach acid has a high disinfecting effect, which can equate us to scavengers. Our stomach contains enzymes designed to digest amino acids that are only in meat. But if we return to raw meat, our stomach actually doesn't like it much, but there's a nuance. If we look at this issue from an evolutionary standpoint, the species Homo sapiens, which we are, is approximately 250,000 years old. The first mentions of the use of fire by primitive people date back to about 1 million years ago. And mass use of fire in everyday life, as numerous excavations show, began around 400,000 years ago. From this, we can assume that our species almost didn't consume raw meat and, as a result, most likely lost the ability to handle raw meat well due to the absence of such a necessity.

There's also a claim that our jaw is adapted only for soft plant food. If you look at the actual set of teeth in our mouth, it's completely universal. We have incisors (for cutting food), canines (like predators, for holding and tearing food), and molars (like herbivores, for chewing), which indicates our adaptation to omnivory. But proponents of diets without meat have an interesting argument. If you actually take a rabbit and try to tear its skin with your teeth (there are many videos with similar experiments), we don't have enough jaw strength for this, making the process of consuming raw meat extremely labor-intensive. And that's true. But as already mentioned, we underwent an evolutionary process for consuming processed meat. This concerns fire, and we can also add sharp stones used to divide the prey. The oldest finds of stone tools date back to 2.5 to 3.0 million years old. Also, if you look at our ancestors, almost all of them have jaws much more massive than ours. For example, Neanderthals, who actually existed parallel to our species (230,000–27,000 years BCE), have a jaw approximately 35% larger than ours, larger muscle attachments, and bones that are significantly thicker. And since muscle strength can increase disproportionately to size, we can assume that not only a rabbit's skin but even your leg could be a fairly achievable target for them.

Based on all that I've written, I conclude for myself that we are omnivores, and all types of calories should be present in our diet. The question is only in the quantity and quality of the food consumed. I definitely wouldn't recommend anyone exclude animal-based food from their diet before the age of 25. Our brain finishes its formation at 25, and a deficiency of certain categories of macronutrients can have a very negative impact on its development, especially in children. The only period, in my opinion, when a diet without meat may make sense for health is the period of the body's maturity when sexual activity is coming to an end. After 60 years, all processes in the body gradually begin to slow down, so theoretically, a lighter diet may make sense. But this isn't certain.

Fasting

Longevity isn't associated with a large number of calories. Those people who constantly consume the conditional norm or even slightly fewer calories than considered necessary live longer in most cases than those who eat even a little more than necessary. There are studies that indirectly show that a slight reduction in caloric intake leads to a potential increase in lifespan. In one study, reducing caloric intake by about 12% over 2 years showed improvements in overall health and cardiovascular system in people[19]. Another study on primates conducted over 25 years specifically confirmed the effect of increased lifespan and higher health levels in monkeys with calorie deficits (25 years of life in monkeys without restrictions versus 32 years in monkeys with deficits)[20].

If we generalize, there are many different similar studies, and most of them prove the benefits of a slight calorie deficit (reducing daily caloric intake by 200–400 calories from the generally established norm). If you look at all this from a logical standpoint, it seems to be true. Personally, I believe that each of us has our internal resource, and a calorie deficit essentially helps slightly reduce the speed of its use.

Invictus Equilibrium

We sort of slow down the burning of our body by adding fewer logs to our furnace. The question is only in the pace of your life. Will you have enough of the reduced number of calories? Before the age of 25, there's probably not much sense in experimenting with this since the body and brain are not yet fully formed. But after 25, it may make sense because, with today's pace of life and energy expenditure needs, a reduced number of calories may actually be sufficient for most people. And don't forget that our body is super adaptive, and positive effects may also be associated with increased efficiency of our energy systems.

It's also scientifically proven that short periods of fasting from 14 to 23 hours can help well in overcoming obesity problems, increasing growth hormone levels, reducing insulin resistance, and effectively helping in the treatment of type 2 diabetes. Intermittent fasting also promotes the activation of longevity genes[21,22,23]. Wikipedia also states that intermittent fasting promotes autophagy, that is, the cleansing and restoration of cells at the molecular level. From what I know, this effect is currently confirmed only in yeast. But in theory, this effect may work in humans.

Our body has many different protective and restorative mechanisms. It's definitely proven that elevated body temperature is a protective mechanism that helps the body fight pathogens. But we also all know that when you're sick, your appetite often disappears, which may indicate that this is also one of the body's protective mechanisms. Therefore, I believe that although the theory of autophagy hasn't been proven in humans yet, there are all reasons to believe that it works. During fasting, our body has time and motivation to focus on internal problems and find ways to solve them optimally rather than digesting food. Essentially, during fasting, our body will feed on everything that's in your body, and it's very logical that it will start with unimportant or harmful compounds.

There are many different methods of long-term fasting, and in fact, most of them don't have normal scientific confirmation. An EXTREMELY large number of books have been written about fasting and its healing properties, but you need to understand that 90% of those books aren't backed by normal scientific research. I don't want to say that fasting doesn't work. I just want to warn everyone against thoughtless self-treatment.

If you look at fasting from an evolutionary standpoint, as I wrote earlier, we're likely well adapted to hunger. If there are no stomach problems, a 48-hour fast shouldn't harm anyone over 25 years old. Fasting is definitely not recommended for children. This can actually harm them quite a bit from my point of view. I personally periodically fast for 36–40 hours. Once every few months, I may have minor

Invictus Equilibrium

disruptions in stomach function, and short-term fasting copes perfectly with everything. For me, it's like rebooting the body.

Anything over 16 hours without calories can already be considered fasting, and if you decide to try, it's better not to practice long fasting immediately. Gradually let your body understand what it's dealing with. You need to realize that the body needs to be prepared for fasting longer than 36 hours. During prolonged fasting, your stomach stops, and the body's overall functioning is reorganized, so it's very important to gradually enter fasting and then gradually exit it. An adequate scheme is when you don't eat heavy food before fasting, and you exit fasting for at least half the time you were fasting. That is, if you fasted for 7 days, then you need about 4 days to gradually increase the number of calories you consume to return to normal nutrition. If you eat well immediately after ending prolonged fasting, it may be your last meal in life.

If you decide to practice fasting, approach this practice with full seriousness and study the issue well. This practice can also have a strong psychological impact. Realizing that you can go without food, for example, for 7 days can significantly boost your confidence.

We, as animals, have a survival instinct, and hunger is one of the best mechanisms that enhances it. "That which does not kill us makes us stronger," as Friedrich Nietzsche once wrote. And there's another wonderful saying by Socrates:

"Hunger is the best seasoning for food." Studies on mice confirm this[24]. And this applies not only to food. If your life is oversaturated with emotions and it's become routine, then "fasting" a bit from movies, phones, showers, sex, etc., can bring back some taste to life.

Microplastics

When talking about nutrition, it's definitely worth mentioning microplastics (these are tiny plastic particles up to 5 microns). Today's world is overflowing with plastic, and it surrounds us everywhere. Plastic greatly simplifies our lives, but unfortunately, we should give it up, and this is a very important step if you care about your future. I won't talk here about the harm of plastic waste to nature (it's actually enormous). We'll only talk about the harm of microplastics to the body.

There are different types of plastic. To simplify, food-grade plastic is divided into disposable and reusable. Most people perceive all plastic as reusable. Few people know, but most plastic water bottles are considered disposable, and reusing them is harmful. But in fact, everything is much worse. Studies prove that two hours of water being in a plastic bottle in the sun saturates it with harmful compounds from the plastic[25]. And that's just two hours. By standards, there's food-grade plastic, and food containers are made from it, for example. But in fact, no one will protect you from mechanical damage to the plastic, and its entry into your body will definitely happen (when you scrape a fork on the container, you're definitely removing a small surface layer).

It's also worth noting that in today's world, zero isn't the norm. This means that a certain amount of micro- or nanoplastic can get into food, but it's considered that this amount is harmless because some studies over a few months have proven that there's no negative impact. But what will happen to your body in 10–20 years is a big question. In my understanding, it's necessary to clearly realize the conditionality of current norms in everything. In fact, our body can overcome an extremely large number of various harmful external influences, but at what cost? Your life resource is definitely not infinite. The fact that you didn't experience any side effects today doesn't mean you didn't spend your life energy and won't have problems in the long term. As my friend says about alcohol: "Drinking today means borrowing mood from tomorrow."

Microplastics can penetrate all organs of our body. Its residues are found even in the blood. It's proven that it can increase the risk of cancer and provoke infertility in both sexes[26,27,28,29]. There are studies proving that consuming drinking water from plastic can lead to an increase in the body's level of female sex hormones and, as a result, to a decrease in testosterone in men[30,31]. And these are definitely not all the already identified side effects of microplastics entering our bodies. Considering all this, I would definitely recommend everyone try to minimize the use of any plastic in their lives. And this especially applies to everything related to nutrition.

Excess Weight

There are a very large number of different methods that contribute to reducing excess weight. Some suggest not eating meat, others to eat only vegetables, etc., but in my opinion, almost always the emphasis is placed on secondary things, completely forgetting about the basics.

The most important thing in any weight loss method is maintaining the balance of energy received and expended. It doesn't matter what you eat (here, the example is specifically about losing weight, not about proper nutrition) and how many calories you consume per day. If you expend more energy than you receive, your weight will decrease. And that's the whole secret! All you need to do to reduce weight is gradually shift the balance of energy expended and received toward a slight deficit.

All this sounds very simple. In practice, it's a bit more complicated. But everything can be achieved if you approach the process wisely. I've already written that all processes

Invictus Equilibrium

occur in our heads. This sounds atypical, but the first thing to realize is that you need to change not your body but your brain, and the body will change itself. To be more precise, you need to make it so that the brain doesn't notice that something has changed, but in fact, you need to change everything.

Our brain is extremely good at associating cause and effect, and it's not always to our benefit. Let's imagine you consume 3,000 kcal per day. And suddenly you decide that it's worth getting ready for summer and go on a diet with 1,500 kcal per day. What does your brain think? "Everything is great; I'm getting ready for summer." Absolutely not! It thinks that a famine year has come. Everything is bad! It tightens absolutely all processes in the body. Cortisol rises to incredible levels, dopamine and serotonin drop. And your brain makes a very simple conclusion: "It was good. Started eating less—it became very bad. So I need to eat more." What's the result? If you didn't last long, you'll only get a clear reinforcement in your brain that dieting is bad, and it won't be easy to start again in the near future. If you lasted longer than a week or a few, lost some weight, and returned to your old diet, you're highly likely to gain more weight than before the diet. This happens because you created an artificial deficit, but the brain perceived it as a real deficit and made an absolutely logical conclusion. If the deficit repeats, you need to be prepared for it, so you need to increase energy reserves in the body.

In my opinion, the best diet option is a balanced diet (the Mediterranean diet is also a very good option), oriented toward products from your region plus sports, but it's extremely important to very carefully introduce your mind and body to such a regimen. It doesn't matter which type of nutrition you choose for yourself. What's important is that everything happens without abrupt changes. You need to gradually reduce the number of calories in your diet, carefully replace bad products with good ones, and gradually add physical activity. If the weight loss process has started, it makes sense to stick to the actual regimen to better form habits for the brain. When the weight stops decreasing, then continue changing the regimen if your goal wasn't achieved in the previous one.

The main guideline, in my opinion, should be cortisol levels. To simplify, you need to make sure your brain doesn't experience great stress at any stage of your transformation. Yes, it will take a long time. In the first period, your progress will be measured in 1–2 kg per month. And I think that's absolutely normal. It's extremely difficult to change in a week what you've been essentially moving toward for half your life (everyone has their own situation, but you should understand the essence). It doesn't matter how small your steps are; what's

Invictus Equilibrium

important is how many you can take. Abusing your nervous system will rarely lead you to the desired result. Just gradually change the conditions, and everything will change.

There's also very interesting information about dishes. It's proven that more food is eaten from large dishes than from small ones. There's an illusion that there's little food on a large plate and a lot on a small one with the same actual amount. From a large plate, 41% more is eaten than from a small one[32]. Also, bright colored dishes (yellow, red, green) increase appetite and, as a result, the amount eaten. On the contrary, dark dishes (dark blue, brown, black) reduce appetite. White can be considered neutral. It doesn't provoke appetite but can highlight the color of the food.

Here's another simple life hack. And for many, this will be the best diet without sports and dietary restrictions. You just need to chew all food 25–30 times. That's not little. But if you do this disciplinedly, only well-chewed food will always enter your stomach, which will be easily digested. And you'll feel satiated with less food. It all works so that you need to feed not the stomach but the brain. It decides when enough is enough. And the satiety signal comes with a delay. Therefore, if you chew food longer and more thoroughly, by the time your brain realizes you've had enough, you'll have eaten less. In fact, it's best to start a diet with this. It really works.

You can also try to fight excess weight by changing the microbiome. Not so long ago, in certain groups of people (mainly in thin ones), a bacterium called Akkermansia muciniphila was found in the microbiome. And there are studies proving that this bacterium plays an important role in maintaining metabolic processes, increases insulin sensitivity (helps with diabetes), and contributes to weight loss[33,34,35]. It's not a magic pill, but it's something that can speed up the weight loss process and possibly even with significant positive additional effects. It can be purchased in the form of supplements and costs reasonable money.

Chapter 12

Stimulants

"True energy is born from within, not from outside."

Mahatma Gandhi

Evolutionarily, it has turned out that we are all oriented toward pleasure. A significant part of our lives is governed by the reward system in our brains. There are many different stimulants, but addictions mainly form from things that bring us pleasure. Our bodies can synthesize various types of their own drugs, and sometimes they indulge us with them. This can enhance pleasure, like when you fall in love, or provide pain relief during injuries. When you consume any stimulants from outside, you disrupt your basic pleasure system, and even after the first time, an addiction begins to form.

How do stimulants and drugs work in general? Our bodies have many different receptors for various substances.

For example, in the reward system area of our brain, there are many nicotine receptors, and our body can also synthesize nicotine. Nicotine actually gives us pleasure and relaxes our nervous system, but there are a few problems. Suppose you have 100 nicotine receptors, and they are set for 1 gram of nicotine per day. When you smoke a cigarette, a dose several times higher than your maximum daily norm of nicotine enters your body at once, giving you a small burst of pleasure. And this is where addiction begins to form.

There are two types of addiction: psychological and physical. Psychological addiction forms immediately. Even after the first puff, your brain clearly remembers the pleasant state you entered; it very well associates cause and effect. And it seems that everything is fine - you smoke and get pleasure. But this won't last long. If large doses of nicotine constantly enter your body, it will quickly begin to adapt. It's not obvious, but the number of receptors will increase (because a lot of nicotine is entering and needs to be processed somehow), but the sensitivity of these receptors will greatly decrease along with the internal synthesis of nicotine. And at moments when nicotine doesn't enter the body from outside, physical withdrawal symptoms begin. All stimulants work on a similar principle. You receive some additional effect that overstimulates your nervous system, and after that, you experience a decline no less in magnitude than the rise, and sometimes even greater. As a result, the physical and psychological desire to get a new dose of emotions increases.

It's important to understand that stimulants without addiction do not exist. All discussions and studies claiming that marijuana or even tea and coffee do not cause addiction are pure data manipulation. There are stimulants that almost do not cause physical dependence, but all of them cause psychological dependence (exceptions may occur in people with psychological disorders). Our brain remembers everything. Any pleasure you received will be associated with something and will remain in your mind forever. The same can be said about fears. If you fell from a tree in childhood, got scared, and reinforced it with pain, the next time you're at a height, the body will preemptively release neurotransmitters of fear to avoid repeating the situation. If you fell and didn't get seriously injured, an illusion of safety may form. And again, we come to the realization of balance.

All stimulants and drugs have positive and negative effects. It's important to clearly understand that any substance on this planet can have positive effects, and this can be easily manipulated. If, for example, someone has cancer and is predicted to have a maximum of two years to live, radiation will be extremely beneficial because it will give them the opportunity to live five, ten, or maybe more years. But if you start irradiating everyone indiscriminately, you understand what will happen. There are many studies that actually prove the benefits of wine, marijuana, hard drugs in small doses, etc. And all those studies are not lying; they just don't investigate the multitude of negative effects that accompany the one positive.

When it comes to the now very fashionable movement of microdosing, I am skeptical about it. But there are nuances. If we consider our evolutionary development, we can assume that stimulants were not present in the lives of our ancestors. Our ancient ancestors could sometimes chew tobacco leaves, for example, or consume something similar, but it was not systematic and always in an unconcentrated form. Therefore, we do not observe any widespread evolutionary adaptations to toxic substances. There are people with congenital immunity to certain poisons, but those are stories about small groups of people and the special conditions of their environment. In general, microdosing is an attempt to get the maximum beneficial effects (mainly to enhance brain function) with minimal harm. Personally, I believe that our body is capable of everything on its own if you learn to feel it, do not interfere with it, and provide it with a sufficient amount of nutrients. This idea is vividly depicted in the film "Limitless." But there are situations in which microdosing certain groups of psychotropics may be appropriate, in my opinion. If you really have genetic deviations related to receptor sensitivity, synthesis of certain neurotransmitters, or psychological problems that truly prevent you from restoring the normal functioning of your nervous system, then perhaps very careful microdosing makes sense. But that's not my path. Drugs are harmful in any doses.

Alcohol

Any amount of alcohol is harmful to our body, and first of all, to the brain. Alcohol physically kills your neurons. There is simply no safe dose, and many different studies prove this[1,2,3]. This could suffice, but it's worth writing a bit about its mechanisms of action because it is one of the most widespread legal drugs in the world.

Alcohol directly damages your brain. To simplify, after alcohol enters the bloodstream, it begins to remove the fatty film from your blood cells (erythrocytes), and they start to stick together, clogging the smallest blood vessels. After starting to drink, most people often have a red nose, ears, and cheeks because there are many very thin vessels there that are the first to clog. But the biggest problem is that there are also many very thin vessels in our brain that get clogged. As a result, most of the brain cells that received oxygen from these vessels simply die and are then excreted from the body along with urine. That is, after a party, in the morning, you literally flush your brain down the toilet. Alcohol in any doses directly leads to a decrease in your brain mass and cognitive dullness. Full recovery of the brain after absolute abstinence from alcohol can take several years. But as a result, you will have a much clearer and more productive mind compared to what you had.

It so happened that I haven't consumed alcohol for more than 14 years, and after many years of observation, I have certain thoughts about why people consume it at all. Scientifically, physical alcohol dependence may not form in everyone. Alcohol addiction develops quite smoothly and slowly. But still, people get hooked on this drug, and I see many social and psychological reasons for this. Alcohol actually relaxes the body and can make us more cheerful, but in essence, it immerses us in psychological states that we can achieve without it. That is, the entire spectrum of emotions you feel under the influence of alcohol can be experienced without it; it's just that some internal, often psychological, barrier stops you. For example, there are many people who are not very good at making new acquaintances, but under the influence of alcohol, they succeed. That is, alcohol simply removes the psychological barrier and helps you be yourself. And it's like that for almost everyone. People look for solutions to their problems in alcohol (the inability to relax and have fun is also a psychological problem). But in fact, alcohol does not solve your problem. It just masks it for a while at the cost of your health and mental abilities. And in the future, you will have an even bigger unresolved psychological problem, compounded by health issues resulting from regular alcohol consumption. Understand the reasons and solve them. Alcohol is harmful!

Nicotine

Smoking is not very good for health. On average, smokers live 14 years less than non-smokers. Just think about how much you'd be willing to pay for an extra 14 years of life. And all you need to do is quit smoking if you smoke. I have sufficiently described the mechanism of nicotine addiction, but here I want to add some data on how to quit if such a problem exists.

Getting rid of physical dependence is relatively simple. On average, the sensitivity of the receptors that respond to nicotine is fully restored in 21 days. It turns out that if you endure 21 days (it's not easy but very possible), only psychological dependence will remain. Overcoming psychological dependence is a bit more difficult. It is much stronger than physical, and it's hard to give advice here because I've never had nicotine dependence. But I have some thoughts. I think that quitting smoking abruptly is not a very good idea for most people. With a sudden cessation, a clear conclusion may form in your mind that it was good before, and when you quit smoking, things became very bad, which can increase psychological pressure. But if you gradually reduce the amount of nicotine and slowly restore receptor sensitivity, the final step of quitting will be very smooth, and the brain won't be able to draw clear conclusions. Everything was normal, you quit, and almost nothing changed.

It's also worth noting that statistics are definitely against you. According to various data, only about 3% to 5% actually quit smoking. One effective method may be replacing the positive emotions from smoking with others in your mind. Remember how good you felt when you didn't smoke. Various breathing practices can also help, such as the Wim Hof Method. They will add oxygen to your body and increase your energy levels. To quit smoking, you really need to rethink the harm this habit brings to your body—how much you're actually losing. Engage in sports and visibly show yourself and your brain the damage smoking has already caused you. Even after a short run, it will be difficult to gather your thoughts while gasping for breath. A great option is to set a fitness goal for yourself. For example, aim to run a marathon in a year or two (42 km is not as easy as it seems), starting your training with 2–5 km and constantly increasing the pace. If you can achieve this, your willpower and self-confidence will skyrocket. You will definitely change forever. Meditation, standing on nails (currently popular "Sadhu Boards"), and stretching can also be good options to ease the fight against addiction. There's also a study showing that the method described in Allen Carr's book "The Easy Way to Stop Smoking" is as effective as nicotine replacement therapy[4].

Relapses are possible, and your task is to constantly increase the intervals between them if you cannot quit immediately. Train your willpower. If you bought a pack of cigarettes, throw it away immediately without hesitation as soon as you realize you're on the wrong path. After quitting, it would also be good to think about helping your body recover with the help of supplements.

No matter how you give it up, your life will definitely change. Once, a friend of my grandfather, in his old age, quit smoking (he had more than 40 years of smoking experience). And I heard an extraordinary phrase from him: "This world has an incredible smell. I really forgot how beautifully tulips smell."

The best way to quit smoking is not to start. Therefore, I think it's worth sharing some effective methods from my grandfathers on how to show your children that smoking is bad so they learn the lesson well. One of my grandfathers, a long time ago, when he found out that my father started smoking, made him eat several cigarettes. I don't know how many cigarettes my father ate at the age of 8, but he still doesn't smoke. This method is not very humane, and modern society may not approve of it, but there's another method from my other grandfather, which I consider the best. When your child first shows interest in cigarettes, don't forbid them from trying; just teach them how to do it correctly. Give your child a cigarette and tell them that they should exhale as much as possible and inhale the cigarette smoke with all their might. This may look a bit harsh; your child will cough for a long time and feel really uncomfortable, but a clear negative association will form in their mind. After that, their friends' talk about how pleasant it is will just be empty words. The main thing is not to miss the moment so that someone else doesn't teach your child to smoke before you. But I think it's definitely not worth teaching before the age of 7.

Coffee, Tea, and Music

Coffee, tea, and music are also stimulants. If I'm wrong, then why can't you easily give them up? Because they affect your body and psyche and lead to pleasant sensations. I grouped these somewhat different stimulants together because most do not consider them stimulants, and they are somewhat similar in their effects. Each of these stimulants excites your nervous system and can cause dependencies, albeit not very strong ones.

Evolutionarily, coffee, tea, and music were not present in primitive people's lives. For millions of years, we drank water and listened only to the sounds of nature. You can find many studies showing the benefits of these stimulants and just as many studies highlighting their harm. An entire book could be written about this, so I will skip all that and convey the main idea about these stimulants.

It can be said for sure that coffee, tea, and music affect our bodies, but if you use these stimulants constantly, their effect will greatly decrease (the development of tolerance to caffeine has been repeatedly proven) and can lead to negative consequences. My main point is that since these stimulants are essentially mild drugs, it's worth perceiving them as cheat codes in your life. If you genuinely lack energy and drink a cup of coffee for the first time in two months, for example, you'll get a maximally strong effect from it, which will definitely outweigh any potential harm. If you have a real need to calm down, a soothing tea will work wonderfully.

Music can also significantly influence our mood. Calm music soothes, while fast-paced music excites our nervous system and can speed us up. You really underestimate its impact. If you are, for example, an athlete and select one song (or melody) that strongly motivates you or helps you concentrate, and you listen to this song only before important competitions, then this song will immerse you as much as possible into the right psychological state. But if you use all these stimulants without particular reason, you greatly reduce their potentially positive effects on your body and disrupt your psyche with endless stimuli that aren't supported by actions. You drink coffee, rev up your body, and sit still. And what does that make you in the eyes of your brain?

Medications

There's definitely no need to write extensively about how the development of medicine has improved our lives and how many lives have been saved. That's all true. There's not much bad in medicine, but in my opinion, people today rely too heavily on conventional treatments and completely forget that their bodies have an extremely large number of defense mechanisms that work perfectly if you don't interfere with them. For example, when we get sick, our body temperature rises, which we try to lower by all means, but in fact, elevated temperature is a defense mechanism. During a fever, most viruses and bacteria die, and our immune system works faster.

My personal philosophy is this: if your body is capable of overcoming an illness on its own without pushing you into

Invictus Equilibrium

critical states, then you don't need to interfere with it using medications. Don't overload your body during illness with heavy food, give yourself rest, drink plenty of water, and your body is capable of overcoming most illnesses on its own. And as a reward, you'll gain stronger immunity.

Don't forget that certain categories of medications can cause dependencies. A vivid example is nasal drops. Most of them form a persistent dependence and can even lead to negative changes in the brain. It's also worth mentioning antibiotics in general. The discovery of antibiotics was groundbreaking in its time and actually saved hundreds of millions of people. But everyone should clearly understand that our body adapts well to everything, and with frequent use of antibiotics, resistance to them develops. They simply stop working. So think carefully when you're recommended to use antibiotics for a common cold. There may come a time when you genuinely need their effect, and they just won't work.

It's also necessary to mention the very common painkillers nowadays. There's nothing terribly bad in the occasional use of painkillers. It's problematic when you ignore the signals of your body. Pain is, first and foremost, a signal of a certain problem.

In general, frequently solving bodily problems with the help of various auxiliary medical means can have negative consequences. Try not to find crutches that temporarily mask the problem but solve the issue comprehensively by finding the cause and eliminating it. If you have a headache, taking painkillers will reduce the pain but won't solve the cause. Make efforts to find the real cause of the pain as soon as possible, and the need for painkillers will simply disappear. Because if you don't pay attention to finding the true cause, the consequences won't be pleasant.

Chapter 13
Vitamins and Minerals

"What you eat today determines how you will feel tomorrow."

Jane Goodall

Vitamins and minerals are components of enzymes, and enzymes (or zymes) are proteins that control and accelerate almost all biochemical processes in our body. We should obtain all necessary vitamins and minerals from food. But unfortunately, the actual amount of minerals and vitamins in today's products is much less than we need and significantly less than what was once present in the same products. For example, a study by the University of Texas at Austin analyzed garden crops from 1950 to 1999 and showed that, on average, protein content decreased by 6%, vitamin B2 by 38%, and vitamin C by 20%. According to the same study, the concentration of minerals like Ca, Mg, Fe, Cu, Na, and P decreased from 18% in calcium to 80% in copper[1]. Another study confirms this trend, showing a decrease in concentrations of all major vitamins and minerals from 1940 to 2019 by values ranging from 14% to 81%[2]. There are many such studies, and they all indicate a strong decrease in the concentration of vitamins and minerals. This can actually be explained.

Today's agriculture is focused on crop quantity rather than quality. We must also add that soil fertility is significantly declining, and there are enough studies to prove this[3,4]. The result is logical. The area is the same, the amount of trace elements has decreased, and yields have increased. As a result, the nutritional value of plant-based products decreases multiple times.

Regarding animal products, the situation is slightly better, but there are still small differences in the mineral composition of wild and farmed meat since their diets differ. And that's not the end of it. We must also consider losses during transportation and various food processing methods[5]. As a result, we conclude that for the normal functioning of our bodies in today's world, it is simply necessary to consume additional vitamins and minerals through supplements. If you don't eat properly for a day, you feel a loss of energy. Now imagine that your body has been undernourished for years. It's very difficult to build anything when you simply don't have the building materials. The state of well-being that you have become accustomed to considering normal is actually just energy-saving. Restoring to a normal level, even with good nutrition using today's products, is a very challenging task and simply impossible for most people. Therefore, additional intake of a controlled amount of vitamins and minerals is the easiest way to buy yourself better well-being and health. In today's world, it is a necessity to simply return your body to normal.

Forms of Vitamins and Minerals

It is quite important to consider the issue of different forms of vitamins and minerals. Regarding vitamins, they can have synthetic or natural origins and be in active or inactive forms. Speaking about synthetic forms, we cannot honestly say that all synthetic forms are worse than natural ones. For example, vitamin B3 is so simple that its synthetic form does not differ from the natural one. Many synthetic forms are simply identical to natural ones or synthesized from natural components, which does not make them worse than pure natural forms. Personally, I have only one question about synthetic forms: how much do I trust the manufacturer? Poorly purified synthetic forms can actually cause harm. Therefore, I personally pay attention to the quality certificates that the manufacturer has. I trust certificates like USP, ConsumerLab, GMP, NSF, UL the most. In general, the presence of any certificate already significantly reduces the likelihood of getting a low-quality supplement. Therefore, if I trust the manufacturer, I see no problems. I buy and monitor how my body perceives this form.

Regarding active and inactive forms, an inactive form is a precursor to the active form, which the body still needs to convert for it to perform its functions. The active form is already converted, and its absorption will be slightly better, but most supplements on the market contain inactive forms that are actually well absorbed by most people. Active forms make sense for those who have digestive problems or genetic poor absorption of a certain vitamin, and inactive forms simply cannot be properly absorbed.

Concerning minerals, minerals in chelated form are absorbed much better. For each mineral molecule in our body to be absorbed, it needs a certain amino acid, enzyme, or protein that will deliver this molecule to the right place. "Chelé" translates from Greek as "claw." That is, the mineral molecule is grabbed in claws and transported to its destination. But since this is not a simple and multi-factorial process, it does not occur with 100% probability, and some of the minerals you consume may simply be excreted without binding. Minerals in chelated form are already bound

Invictus Equilibrium

(chelated), and their absorption in the body will be much higher than ordinary forms.

It should also be said that all this carries a recommendatory character, and in fact, the best form of a vitamin or mineral should be selected individually, and there's no way around self-testing. For example, taking certain forms of zinc, especially in increased dosages, can cause various unpleasant sensations in the stomach. Personally, I used to take 50 milligrams of zinc gluconate (chelated form) 2 times a week, and sometimes it caused slight specific discomfort. But when I started taking 25 milligrams 4 times a week of the same form, all discomfort disappeared. The most common chelated forms are lysinate, monomethionine, aspartate, methionine, glycinate, citrate, acetate, fumarate, gluconate, picolinate, orotate, and others.

It's also important to clearly understand that with dietary supplements (especially concerning dosages much higher than prophylactic), one should still be cautious. An excess of certain vitamins and minerals can sometimes be more harmful than a deficiency. Therefore, thoughtless intake, especially of multivitamins, will not always be beneficial. There is one big problem with multivitamins. Each vitamin has many different forms and structures. For example, vitamin C has at least 6 different forms, and the point is that different forms of different vitamins can be incompatible with each other. It turns out that in a tablet with ten vitamins and minerals, eight can be incompatible and will simply neutralize each other, bringing no benefit, and the rest that remains may be exactly what you already have enough of. Even knowing this, more often taking multivitamins with prophylactic dosages will be better than not taking them, but personally, I chose the option of taking most vitamins and minerals separately. In my opinion, for most vitamins and minerals, it's better to take 300% of the daily norm once every 3–5 days in an individual form than the daily norm all together.

Water-Soluble Vitamins

All vitamins known today are divided into two groups: water-soluble and fat-soluble. As the name implies, some dissolve in water, others in fats. Water-soluble vitamins are directly absorbed into the blood and stay in the body on average from 1 to 3 days. Therefore, they should regularly enter our body. They do not accumulate, and their excess is excreted by the kidneys. Water-soluble vitamins include all B-group vitamins, vitamins C and H.

Invictus Equilibrium

All norms here and further are indicated for men/women aged 19 to 60 years.

Vitamin B₁ (Thiamine, Anti-Neuritic) – participates in cellular respiration.

Symptoms of Possible Deficiency: Nervous system disorders, vision impairment, unsteadiness while walking, confusion, memory loss, exhaustion, loss of appetite, anemia, enlarged heart, tachycardia.

Symptoms of Overdose: Unknown.

Synthetic Forms: Thiamine hydrochloride (bioavailability about 100%), thiamine mononitrate (high bioavailability, about 95%).

Natural Sources: Whole grains, legumes, nuts, lean meat, fish, eggs.

Intake Recommendations: Recommended to take with food for better absorption. Alcohol can reduce thiamine levels, so people who consume alcohol should pay special attention to its intake.

Daily Norm: 1.2 mg/1.1 mg.

Vitamin B$_2$ (Riboflavin, Growth Vitamin) – helps the body produce energy and supports growth, participates in important metabolic processes.

Symptoms of Possible Deficiency: Skin problems (dermatitis), cracks at the corners of the mouth, lips and tongue may become bright red and shiny. Possible eye problems: increased sensitivity to light, blurred vision.

Symptoms of Overdose: Unknown.

Synthetic Forms: Riboflavin-5'-phosphate sodium (bioavailability about 60–70%).

Natural Sources: Dairy products, meat, fish, eggs, green vegetables, whole grains.

Intake Recommendations: Riboflavin should be taken with food, as it improves absorption. It is sensitive to light, so products and supplements should be stored in a dark place.

Daily Norm: 1.3 mg/1.1 mg.

Invictus Equilibrium

Vitamin B$_3$ (Niacin, Nicotinamide, Anti-Pellagra Vitamin) – important for converting food into energy, supports skin health, nervous and digestive systems.

Symptoms of Possible Deficiency: Pellagra, manifested by fatigue, headaches, loss of appetite, dry mouth, nausea, diarrhea, dry skin with ulcers, memory and mood problems.

Symptoms of Overdose: High doses can cause skin flushing, increased blood sugar levels, liver problems. Harmful doses start after 2 g per day.

Synthetic Forms:

- Niacin (Nicotinic Acid): Bioavailability about 88%.
- Niacinamide (Nicotinamide): Bioavailability close to 100%.

Natural Sources: Meat, fish, nuts, legumes, whole grains, some vegetables.

Intake Recommendations: Niacin can be taken with or without food. High doses of niacin can cause skin flushing, so consultation with a doctor is advised when prescribing high doses.

Daily Norm: 16 mg/14 mg.

Vitamin B$_5$ (Pantothenic Acid, Anti-Dermatitis Vitamin) – necessary for energy production, synthesis of fats, hormones, and red blood cells.

Symptoms of Possible Deficiency: Rare, may include loss of appetite, fatigue, numbness or tingling in hands and feet.

Symptoms of Overdose: Unknown.

Synthetic Forms: Calcium pantothenate, sodium pantothenate (bioavailability about 50%).

Natural Sources: Meat, eggs, whole grains, legumes, avocado, broccoli.

Intake Recommendations: Pantothenic acid is recommended to be taken with food. Deficiency is rare since the vitamin is widely available in foods.

Daily Norm: 5 mg/5 mg.

Invictus Equilibrium

Vitamin B₆ (Pyridoxine, Anti-Dermatitis Vitamin) – important for amino acid metabolism, formation of red blood cells and antibodies, supports the nervous system.

Symptoms of Possible Deficiency: In children: irritability, seizures, anemia, vomiting. In adults: skin problems around the eyes and mouth, increased risk of heart disease.

Symptoms of Overdose: Numbness of limbs, difficulty walking, nerve damage. Harmful dose starts from 100 mg per day.

Synthetic Forms: Pyridoxine hydrochloride (bioavailability about 75%).

Natural Sources: Meat, poultry, fish, bananas, nuts, whole grains, vegetables.

Intake Recommendations: Take with food for better absorption. Some medications can reduce vitamin B6 levels, so consultation with a doctor may be useful.

Daily Norm: 1.3–1.7 mg/1.2–1.5 mg.

Vitamin B$_9$ (Folic Acid, Anti-Anemia Vitamin) – necessary for DNA formation and new cells, especially important during pregnancy for fetal nervous system development.

Symptoms of Possible Deficiency: Anemia, digestive problems, diarrhea. In newborns, possible congenital neural tube defects.

Symptoms of Overdose: Officially considered unknown, but some studies indicate certain risks with long-term intake of more than 1,000 µg per day. This vitamin can accumulate in the body, forming reserves for several months. Excessive consumption of folic acid can also mask vitamin B$_{12}$ deficiency, which can have unpleasant consequences, especially neurological problems that may sometimes be irreversible.

Synthetic Forms: Folic acid (synthetic form bioavailability about 85% when taken with food, up to 100% on an empty stomach).

Natural Sources: Leafy green vegetables (spinach, broccoli), legumes, citrus fruits, fortified grain products (natural form - folates).

Invictus Equilibrium

Intake Recommendations: Women planning pregnancy or who are pregnant are recommended additional folic acid intake. Folic acid is better taken with food.

<u>Daily Norm:</u> 400 µg/400 µg.

Vitamin B$_{12}$ (Cobalamin, Cyanocobalamin, Anti-Anemia Vitamin) – necessary for the formation of red blood cells, supports nervous system health.

Symptoms of Possible Deficiency: Anemia, pallor, loss of appetite, weight loss, shortness of breath, nervous disorders. Often occurs due to poor absorption rather than lack in diet.

Symptoms of Overdose: Currently unknown. This may be due to its significant accumulation in the liver, kidneys, or other tissues. Accumulated reserves may be sufficient for a period from several months to 5 years.

Synthetic Forms:

- Cyanocobalamin: Common synthetic form with bioavailability about 50%.
- Methylcobalamin: Bioavailability may be higher, about 55%.

Natural Sources: Animal products: meat, fish, dairy products, eggs.

Intake Recommendations: Vegetarians and vegans are recommended additional vitamin B_{12} intake. Take with food. Absorption depends on the presence of "intrinsic factor" in the stomach.

<u>*Daily Norm:*</u> 2.4 µg/2.4 µg.

Vitamin H (B_7, Biotin, Anti-Seborrheic Vitamin) – helps in the metabolism of fats and amino acids, important for healthy skin, hair, and nails.

Symptoms of Possible Deficiency: Dry skin, brittle hair, muscle pain, fatigue, loss of appetite.

Symptoms of Overdose: Unknown.

Synthetic Forms: D-Biotin (synthetic form, bioavailability close to 100%).

Natural Sources: Eggs (especially yolk), liver, nuts, soy, cauliflower.

Invictus Equilibrium

Intake Recommendations: Biotin can be taken with or without food. Long-term consumption of raw egg whites can reduce biotin absorption.

Daily Norm: 30 µg/30 µg.

Vitamin C (Ascorbic Acid, Anti-Scurvy Vitamin) – powerful antioxidant, necessary for collagen synthesis, strengthens the immune system, improves iron absorption.

Symptoms of Possible Deficiency: Scurvy: weakness, joint pain, dental problems, slow wound healing, bleeding gums, anemia.

Symptoms of Overdose: Large doses (10 times or more than the recommendation) can cause diarrhea, kidney stone formation.

Synthetic Forms: Ascorbic acid (bioavailability of synthetic and natural forms is approximately the same, about 70–90% at doses up to 180 mg per day).

Natural Sources: Citrus fruits, berries, kiwi, broccoli, bell peppers.

Intake Recommendations: Vitamin C can be taken with or without food. Higher doses (over 1 g) may have reduced bioavailability and may cause gastrointestinal discomfort. It should also be noted that vitamin C is quite actively destroyed during thermal processing, in light, and upon contact with metals.

Daily Norm: 90 mg/75 mg.

Fat-Soluble Vitamins

While water-soluble vitamins can be taken without monitoring and simply taken in prophylactic doses, it's a bit different with fat-soluble vitamins. They accumulate in adipose tissue and can have toxic effects when excessively accumulated. Their levels are better controlled by periodically taking tests and adjusting dosages based on them. Fat-soluble vitamins include vitamins A, E, D, and K.

Vitamin A (Retinol, Anti-Xerophthalmic Vitamin) – important for eye health, supports good vision, especially in low light conditions. Also supports skin and mucous membrane health, promotes normal bone and tooth growth, supports reproductive function, and acts as an antioxidant.

Invictus Equilibrium

Symptoms of Possible Deficiency: Night blindness, dry skin and hair, skin and mucous membrane problems, increased susceptibility to infections, dry eyes, corneal clouding. In pregnant women, possible fetal development disorders.

Symptoms of Overdose: Prolonged intake of large doses (more than 10 mg per day for months) can be toxic. Possible nausea, vomiting, loss of appetite, headache, hair loss, joint pain, brittle bones, enlargement of the liver and spleen. In smokers, may increase the risk of lung cancer.

Synthetic Forms: Retinyl acetate, retinyl palmitate (bioavailability about 70–90% when taken with fats).

Natural Forms:

- Retinoids: Liver, fish oil, dairy products, egg yolk.
- Carotenoids (Beta-Carotene): Carrots, sweet potatoes, spinach, apricots (beta-carotene is not equal to vitamin A; 12 units of beta-carotene are converted in the body into ~1 unit of vitamin A).

Intake Recommendations: Since vitamin A is fat-soluble, it should be taken with foods containing fats. Excessive intake of retinol can be toxic, while beta-carotene is considered a safer source.

Daily Norm: 900 µg/700 µg.

Vitamin D (Calciferol, Anti-Rachitic Vitamin) – promotes calcium absorption in the body, helps maintain healthy bones and teeth. Important for proper nervous system function, muscle contractions, and blood clotting.

Symptoms of Possible Deficiency: In children, can lead to rickets (bone development disorders), in adults to osteomalacia (softening of the bones). Possible muscle weakness, leg pain, irritability.

Symptoms of Overdose: High doses can be toxic, especially for children. Symptoms include vomiting, diarrhea, fatigue, weight loss, elevated calcium levels in the blood, calcium deposits in soft tissues, possible irreversible damage to the heart and kidneys.

Synthetic Forms:

- Vitamin D_2 (Ergocalciferol): Bioavailability may be lower than D_3.
- Vitamin D_3 (Cholecalciferol): High bioavailability, considered more effective.

Invictus Equilibrium

Natural Sources: Synthesized in the skin under sunlight exposure. Found in fatty fish, fish oil, egg yolks.

Intake Recommendations: Vitamin D is better taken with foods containing fats. Doses over 4,000 IU per day with prolonged use can be toxic. Absorbed better with sufficient magnesium and vitamin K in the body.

<u>Daily Norm:</u> 15 µg/15 µg.

Vitamin E (Tocopherols, Anti-Sterility Vitamin, Reproduction Vitamin) – acts as an antioxidant, protects cells from damage caused by free radicals. Supports skin, eye, and immune health, may help prevent cardiovascular diseases.

Symptoms of Possible Deficiency: Very rare. May include muscle weakness, coordination problems, nervous system damage, anemia due to destruction of red blood cells.

Symptoms of Overdose: Even at high doses, usually no serious side effects are observed, but they are sometimes possible. Potential overdose symptoms include delayed wound healing, muscle, bone, or joint pain, irritability, persistent nausea, weakness, decreased blood clotting, which can lead to increased bleeding.

Synthetic Forms: DL-alpha-tocopherol (synthetic, bioavailability about 50% of the natural form).

Natural Forms: D-alpha-tocopherol (natural form, high bioavailability), found in vegetable oils, nuts, seeds, avocado.

Intake Recommendations: Vitamin E should be taken with foods containing fats. The synthetic form is less effective, so preference should be given to the natural form. Selenium and vitamin C significantly enhance the absorption efficiency of vitamin E.

Daily Norm: 15 mg/15 mg.

Vitamin K (Naphthoquinones, Anti-Hemorrhagic Vitamin) – necessary for normal blood clotting, helps synthesize proteins involved in this process. Also supports bone health.

Symptoms of Possible Deficiency: Blood clotting problems, prolonged bleeding even with small cuts, easy bruising.

Symptoms of Overdose: Unknown or very rare.

Synthetic Forms: Phytonadione (vitamin K_1, synthetic, bioavailability about 50% when taken with fats).

Natural Forms:

- Vitamin K_1 (Phylloquinone): Green leafy vegetables.
- Vitamin K_2 (Menaquinone): Fermented products, some cheeses, eggs (bioavailability of K_2 may be higher, especially MK-7 forms).

Intake Recommendations: Take with foods containing fats. Vitamin K_2 (especially MK-7) has a longer half-life and may be more effective in maintaining vitamin K levels.

Daily Norm: 120 µg/110 µg.

It's important for the body to have all vitamins. The effectiveness of most increases significantly in symbiosis with other vitamins and minerals. It should also be understood that not all positive effects of different vitamins and minerals have been identified. Each of them has a huge number of benefits unless we are talking about toxic concentrations. For example, vitamin D is associated with at least 2,500 different genes in our body, and we do not yet fully understand the entirety of these reactions. Therefore, it's impossible to accurately diagnose based on certain symptoms and can't rely precisely on norms.

If we generalize the possibility of overdose with fat-soluble vitamins, the dose you take is not so important. What matters is how much vitamin has accumulated in the body overall. If you have a large deficiency determined by test results, then taking dosages that exceed the norm by 10 or 20 times for a certain period will be absolutely rational.

Minerals

Minerals are mineral substances required in varying amounts to ensure the normal functioning of all systems in the body.

Iron (Fe)

Role: Key component of hemoglobin that transports oxygen throughout the body; supports immune and cognitive functions.

Signs of Deficiency: Anemia, fatigue, pale skin, shortness of breath, dizziness, cold extremities.

Signs of Overdose: Iron poisoning, which may cause abdominal pain, nausea, vomiting; in severe cases - organ damage.

Non-Chelated Forms: Iron sulfate (absorption ~10-15%), iron fumarate.

Chelated Forms: Iron bisglycinate (high absorption, up to 90%), iron gluconate.

Natural Forms: Heme iron from meat, liver, fish; non-heme iron from legumes, dark green vegetables, fortified grains.

Recommendations for Intake: Best taken on an empty stomach or between meals for better absorption. Vitamin C enhances iron absorption - can be taken together with citrus fruits or berries. It's advisable to avoid simultaneous intake with calcium, antacids (medications that reduce stomach acidity), tea, or coffee, as they reduce iron absorption.

<u>*Daily Norm:*</u> 8 mg/18 mg.

Iodine (I)

Role: Essential for the synthesis of thyroid hormones that regulate metabolism, growth, and development.

Signs of Deficiency: Goiter (enlarged thyroid gland), hypothyroidism, delayed mental and physical development in children.

Signs of Overdose: Hyperthyroidism, symptoms include weight loss, rapid heartbeat, anxiety.

Non-Chelated Forms: Potassium iodide.

Chelated Forms: Iodine is usually not available in chelated forms.

Natural Forms: Iodine from seaweeds (e.g., kelp), seafood.

Recommendations for Intake: Take during meals for better absorption. Avoid excessive consumption, especially with thyroid disorders. Consultation with a doctor is recommended.

Daily Norm: 150 µg.

Magnesium (Mg)

Role: Participates in over 300 enzymatic reactions, important for nervous and muscular function, supports bone and heart health. Studies have shown that magnesium supplementation leads to a significant reduction in depression symptoms[6,7,8].

Signs of Deficiency: Muscle spasms, heart arrhythmias, anxiety, depression, insomnia.

Signs of Overdose: Diarrhea, nausea, lowered blood pressure; in severe cases—heart failure.

Non-Chelated Forms: Magnesium oxide (absorption ~4%), magnesium sulfate.

Chelated Forms: Magnesium citrate (absorption ~25–30%), magnesium glycinate (up to 80%), magnesium malate.

Natural Forms: Nuts, seeds, dark green leafy vegetables, whole grains.

Recommendations for Intake: Better taken with food to improve absorption and reduce the risk of stomach upset. Evening intake may promote relaxation and improve sleep.

Consuming with grains may worsen absorption. Adequate vitamin B_6 is necessary for normal magnesium absorption.

Daily Norm: 420 mg/320 mg.

Calcium (Ca)

Role: Necessary for healthy bones and teeth, normal muscle function, nervous system activity, and blood clotting.

Signs of Deficiency: Osteoporosis, frequent fractures, muscle spasms, tingling in extremities.

Signs of Overdose: Hypercalcemia, which can lead to kidney stones, nausea, weakness.

Non-Chelated Forms: Calcium carbonate (absorption ~30–40%), calcium phosphate.

Chelated Forms: Calcium citrate (absorption ~35–45%), calcium glycinate.

Natural Forms: Dairy products, dark green leafy vegetables, almonds, sardines with bones.

Recommendations for Intake: Take with food, especially calcium carbonate. Vitamin D enhances calcium absorption, so it's advisable to take them together. Avoid simultaneous intake with iron or zinc and grains.

Daily Norm: 1,000 mg.

Zinc (Zn)

Role: Important for the immune system, normal functioning of the male reproductive system, synthesis of testosterone and growth hormone, wound healing, DNA and protein synthesis; supports taste and smell. Long-term zinc deficiency can lead to erectile dysfunction in men and heart attack.

Signs of Deficiency: Frequent infections, slow wound healing, hair loss, loss of appetite.

Signs of Overdose: Nausea, vomiting, diarrhea, impaired immune function; high doses may cause copper deficiency.

Non-Chelated Forms: Zinc oxide (absorption ~50%), zinc sulfate.

Chelated Forms: Zinc picolinate (absorption ~60–70%), zinc gluconate, zinc bisglycinate.

Natural Forms: Meat, shellfish, whole grains, nuts, seeds.

Recommendations for Intake: Take on an empty stomach or 1–2 hours before meals. If stomach upset occurs, take with food. Absorption may be impaired when taken simultaneously with iron, calcium, copper, and vitamin B_9. Also poorly absorbed with grains.

<u>*Daily Norm:*</u> 11 mg/8 mg.

Selenium (Se)

Role: Antioxidant, supports thyroid function and immune system.

Signs of Deficiency: Muscle weakness, cardiomyopathy, decreased immunity.

Signs of Overdose: Selenosis—hair and nail loss, fatigue, neurological disorders.

Non-Chelated Forms: Sodium selenite.

Chelated Forms: Selenomethionine (high bioavailability).

Invictus Equilibrium

Natural Forms: Brazil nuts, seafood, meat, grains (depends on soil content).

Recommendations for Intake: Take with food. Can be combined with vitamin E to enhance antioxidant effect.

<u>Daily Norm:</u> 55 µg.

Potassium (K)

Role: Important for heart, muscle, and nerve function; regulates fluid and electrolyte balance.

Signs of Deficiency: Muscle weakness, irregular heartbeat, fatigue, cramps.

Signs of Overdose: Hyperkalemia, which can lead to cardiac arrhythmias.

Non-Chelated Forms: Potassium chloride, potassium bicarbonate.

Chelated Forms: Potassium citrate, potassium aspartate.

Natural Forms: Bananas, avocados, potatoes, spinach, legumes.

Recommendations for Intake: Usually obtained adequately from food. If supplementing, take with food.

<u>Daily Norm:</u> 4,700 mg.

Copper (Cu)

Role: Involved in the production of red blood cells, supports nervous and immune systems.

Signs of Deficiency: Anemia, brittle bones, pigmentation disorders of skin and hair.

Signs of Overdose: Nausea, liver and kidney damage.

Non-Chelated Forms: Copper sulfate.

Chelated Forms: Copper gluconate, copper bisglycinate.

Natural Forms: Shellfish, nuts, seeds, whole grain products.

Recommendations for Intake: Take with food. Avoid excessive zinc intake, which can reduce copper absorption and lead to its deficiency. The zinc to copper ratio should be approximately 10:1.

Invictus Equilibrium

Daily Norm: 900 µg.

Chromium (Cr)

Role: Helps regulate blood glucose levels, enhances insulin action.

Signs of Deficiency: Impaired glucose tolerance, increased risk of type 2 diabetes.

Signs of Overdose: Rare; possible kidney and liver problems.

Non-Chelated Forms: Chromium chloride.

Chelated Forms: Chromium picolinate, chromium polynicotinate.

Natural Forms: Broccoli, whole grain products, meat, nuts.

Recommendations for Intake: Take during meals. May be beneficial to take with carbohydrates.

Daily Norm: 35 µg.

Manganese (Mn)

Role: Participates in the metabolism of carbohydrates and amino acids, necessary for bone formation.

Signs of Deficiency: Rare; may include growth disorders, bone deformities.

Signs of Overdose: Neurological symptoms, coordination disorders.

Non-Chelated Forms: Manganese sulfate.

Chelated Forms: Manganese gluconate, manganese bisglycinate.

Natural Forms: Whole grain products, nuts, leafy vegetables, tea.

Recommendations for Intake: Take with food. Avoid excessive intake.

Daily Norm: 2.3 mg/1.8 mg.

Invictus Equilibrium

Molybdenum (Mo)

Role: Involved in the metabolism of amino acids and purines.

Signs of Deficiency: Extremely rare; possible neurological disorders.

Signs of Overdose: May lead to gout.

Non-Chelated Forms: Molybdenum trioxide.

Chelated Forms: Molybdenum glycinate.

Natural Forms: Legumes, grains, nuts.

Recommendations for Intake: Usually does not require additional supplementation. Take with food if prescribed.

<u>Daily Norm:</u> 45 µg.

Phosphorus (P)

Role: Supports bone and teeth health, involved in energy production.

Signs of Deficiency: Weakness, bone pain, anorexia.

Signs of Overdose: Disruption of calcium and phosphorus balance.

Non-Chelated Forms: Dicalcium phosphate.

Chelated Forms: Phosphorus is usually not available in chelated forms.

Natural Forms: Meat, fish, dairy products, nuts.

Recommendations for Intake: Usually adequately obtained from food. Additional supplementation is rarely needed.

Daily Norm: 700 mg.

Sodium (Na)

Role: Maintains fluid and electrolyte balance, necessary for nerve function.

Invictus Equilibrium

Signs of Deficiency: Hyponatremia, causing headaches, nausea, fatigue.

Signs of Overdose: High blood pressure, edema.

Non-Chelated Forms: Sodium chloride (table salt).

Chelated Forms: Sodium does not require chelated forms.

Natural Forms: Salty foods, canned goods.

Recommendations for Intake: Avoid excessive consumption. Usually sufficient from food.

<u>Daily Norm:</u> 1,800 mg.

Chlorine (Cl)

Role: Maintains fluid and electrolyte balance, component of stomach acid.

Signs of Deficiency: Loss of appetite, muscle weakness.

Signs of Overdose: High blood pressure, edema.

Non-Chelated Forms: Sodium chloride.

Chelated Forms: Chlorine is not offered in chelated forms.

Natural Forms: Salty foods, seafood.

Recommendations for Intake: Usually sufficient from food. Avoid excessive consumption.

<u>Daily Norm:</u> 2,300 mg.

Sulfur (S)

Role: Part of amino acids and vitamins, important for skin, hair, and nails.

Signs of Deficiency: Brittle hair and nails, skin problems.

Signs of Overdose: Generally non-toxic; excess is excreted. Possible mild symptoms like diarrhea, headache, rashes, and nausea.

Non-Chelated Forms: Methylsulfonylmethane (MSM).

Invictus Equilibrium

Chelated Forms: Sulfur is not offered in chelated forms.

Natural Forms: Meat, fish, eggs, garlic, onions.

Recommendations for Intake: Usually sufficient from diet. MSM is best taken with food.

<u>Daily Norm:</u> No exact data. Safe dosages are considered to be from 500 mg to 8,000 mg per day divided into 2-3 doses.

Fluorine (F)

Role: Strengthens tooth enamel, prevents dental caries.

Signs of Deficiency: Increased risk of cavities.

Signs of Overdose: Fluorosis - spotting of teeth, bone damage.

Non-Chelated Forms: Sodium fluoride.

Chelated Forms: Fluorine is not available in chelated forms.

Natural Forms: Fluoridated water, tea, seafood.

Recommendations for Intake: Usually obtained from water and toothpaste. Additional supplementation is not needed.

Daily Norm: 2-5 mg.

Cobalt (Co)

Role: Component of vitamin B_{12}, necessary for blood formation.

Signs of Deficiency: Anemia, fatigue, neurological disorders.

Signs of Overdose: Heart problems, thyroid issues.

Non-Chelated Forms: Cobalt chloride.

Chelated Forms: Cobalt gluconate.

Natural Forms: Animal products (through vitamin B_{12}).

Recommendations for Intake: Usually sufficient vitamin B_{12} from food. Additional cobalt supplementation is not needed.

Daily Norm: No established norm. Recommended dose is 7–15 µg.

Vitamin-Like Substances and Provitamins

Since the topics of vitamins and minerals have been thoroughly covered, it's sensible to consider substances that also play a significant role in the normal functioning of the body. Therefore, we will discuss vitamin-like substances and provitamins.

Vitamin-like substances are compounds that are not included in the classical list of vitamins but are very similar to them in biochemical functions and are also quite important for health. Most of them can be synthesized in small quantities by the body, so their additional intake is not mandatory, although it can be beneficial. Vitamin-like substances are not classified as vitamins also because they do not have pronounced deficiency symptoms. If they are not supplied to the body, no sharp changes occur.

Vitamin B₄ (Choline)

Role: Necessary for the synthesis of acetylcholine, a neurotransmitter important for memory and muscle activity. Also involved in fat metabolism and supports liver health.

Symptoms of Possible Deficiency: Fatty liver disease, memory impairment, elevated homocysteine levels, nervous system problems.

Symptoms of Overdose: Unpleasant body odor (fishy smell), sweating, lowered blood pressure, diarrhea, nausea.

Synthetic Forms: Choline chloride, choline bitartrate.

Natural Sources: Egg yolks, liver, meat, fish, legumes, nuts, whole grain products.

Recommendations for Intake: Recommended to consume with food. Especially important for pregnant and breastfeeding women for the baby's brain development.

Daily Norm: 550 mg/400 mg.

Vitamin B₈ (Inositol)

Role: Plays a role in cellular signal transmission, influences fat and insulin metabolism, supports nervous system health.

Symptoms of Possible Deficiency: Depression, anxiety, insomnia, elevated cholesterol levels, skin and hair problems.

Symptoms of Overdose: At high doses, possible nausea, diarrhea, dizziness.

Synthetic Forms: Myo-inositol, D-chiro-inositol.

Natural Sources: Citrus fruits, whole grain products, legumes, nuts, seeds.

Recommendations for Intake: May be beneficial in polycystic ovary syndrome, depression. Intake should be coordinated with a doctor.

Daily Norm: No established official norm; doses in studies vary from 500 mg to 2,000 mg. Wikipedia mentions a norm of 500 mg per day.

Vitamin B₁₀ (Para-Aminobenzoic Acid, PABA)

Role: Involved in the synthesis of folic acid, may support skin and hair health.

Symptoms of Possible Deficiency: Increased sensitivity to sunlight, eczema, hair depigmentation.

Symptoms of Overdose: Nausea, vomiting, impaired liver function at high doses.

Synthetic Forms: PABA in supplement form.

Natural Sources: Liver, yeast, mushrooms, spinach, whole grain products.

Recommendations for Intake: Usually obtained from diet; supplements should be taken after consulting a doctor.

<u>Daily Norm:</u> No established official norm. Unofficial recommendations are about 100 mg per day.

Vitamin B₁₁ (L-Carnitine)

Role: Necessary for transporting fatty acids into mitochondria for energy production. Supports heart and muscle function.

Symptoms of Possible Deficiency: Muscle weakness, fatigue, impaired heart activity.

Symptoms of Overdose: Nausea, diarrhea, possible fishy body odor at high doses.

Synthetic Forms: L-carnitine, acetyl-L-carnitine.

Natural Sources: Red meat, fish, poultry, dairy products.

Recommendations for Intake: May be beneficial for athletes and people with cardiovascular diseases. Intake should be coordinated with a doctor.

<u>*Daily Norm:*</u> No established official norm; studies use doses from 300 mg to 2,000 mg. Dosage varies greatly depending on physical activity. Recommendations of up to 3,000 mg are found for athletes.

Vitamin B_{13} (Orotic Acid)

Role: Involved in the synthesis of nucleic acids (DNA and RNA), supports the metabolism of folic acid and vitamin B12.

Symptoms of Possible Deficiency: Not established in humans.

Symptoms of Overdose: Digestive disorders at high doses.

Synthetic Forms: Mineral orotates (e.g., magnesium orotate).

Natural Sources: Dairy products, brewer's yeast, root vegetables.

Recommendations for Intake: Usually adequately obtained from diet but may be beneficial when there's a need to accelerate liver cell regeneration, helps reduce cholesterol levels, and positively affects reproductive function and growth processes (particularly muscle tissue).

<u>Daily Norm:</u> No established official norm, but depending on physical activity levels, recommendations range from 500 mg to 3,000 mg.

Vitamin B$_{14}$ (Pyrroloquinoline Quinone, PQQ)

Role: A compound sometimes referred to as vitamin B14 in some sources but not officially recognized as a

Invictus Equilibrium

vitamin. PQQ has antioxidant properties, supports mitochondrial function, and may promote neuroprotection and the growth of new mitochondria. Some data consider it the most potent antioxidant. There's a concept of antioxidant recycling, i.e., how many cycles an antioxidant can go through without losing its properties. For vitamin C, it's about 4 cycles; for PQQ, it's 20,000 cycles.

Symptoms of Possible Deficiency: No established deficiency symptoms in humans, as it's not recognized as an essential nutrient for humans.

Symptoms of Overdose: Data on toxicity and overdose symptoms in humans are limited. At high doses, possible gastrointestinal disturbances, insomnia, headache.

Synthetic Forms: Pyrroloquinoline quinone is available as a dietary supplement.

Natural Sources: Natto (fermented soybeans), green peppers, parsley, kiwi, papaya, green tea, spinach.

Recommendations for Intake: No established official recommendations for daily PQQ intake.

<u>Daily Norm:</u> No established official daily intake norm for PQQ. Various recommendations suggest a

potentially beneficial dose ranging between 5 mg and 40 mg per day.

Vitamin B$_{15}$ (Pangamic Acid)

Role: Attributed with antioxidant properties, supports metabolism and detoxification.

Symptoms of Possible Deficiency: Not established in humans.

Symptoms of Overdose: Possible headache, nausea at high doses.

Synthetic Forms: Calcium pangamate.

Natural Sources: Apricot kernels, whole grain products, seeds, nuts.

Recommendations for Intake: Not officially recognized as a vitamin in many countries but is used for treating atherosclerosis, chronic coronary insufficiency, and chronic hepatitis.

<u>Daily Norm:</u> No established official norm. Therapeutic doses are considered to be from 100 mg to 300

mg per day.

Lipoic Acid (Vitamin N)

Role: A potent antioxidant, involved in energy metabolism, improves insulin sensitivity.

Symptoms of Possible Deficiency: Rare, as the body synthesizes it independently.

Symptoms of Overdose: Possible skin rashes, hypoglycemia at high doses.

Synthetic Forms: Alpha-lipoic acid.

Natural Sources: Spinach, broccoli, meat, liver, yeast.

Recommendations for Intake: Used in diabetes and neuropathy. Has shown high effectiveness in treating various chronic hepatitis, liver cirrhosis, and various poisonings and intoxications, even with heavy metal salts.

<u>*Daily Norm:*</u> No official norm. Usually 300–600 mg for therapeutic purposes.

Coenzyme Q10 (Ubiquinone)

Role: Important for energy production in cells, has antioxidant properties, supports the cardiovascular system.

Symptoms of Possible Deficiency: Fatigue, muscle weakness, heart problems.

Symptoms of Overdose: Nausea, diarrhea, loss of appetite at high doses.

Synthetic Forms: Coenzyme Q10 in ubiquinone and ubiquinol forms.

Natural Sources: Red meat, fatty fish, nuts, seeds.

Recommendations for Intake: Take with foods containing fats for better absorption. May be beneficial for people taking statins.

Daily Norm: No official norm. Recommended dose may vary from 30 mg to 200 mg depending on physical activity.

Invictus Equilibrium

Bioflavonoids (Vitamin P)

Role: A group of antioxidants that enhance the action of vitamin C, support the health of blood vessels and capillaries by exhibiting anti-inflammatory and capillary-strengthening effects.

Symptoms of Possible Deficiency: Easy bruising, nosebleeds, swelling.

Symptoms of Overdose: Generally safe, but at high doses, allergic reactions are possible.

Synthetic Forms: Rutin, hesperidin.

Natural Sources: Citrus fruits, berries, buckwheat, green tea, red wine.

Recommendations for Intake: Consume during meals, but it's better to obtain from diet. Used in hemorrhagic diathesis and peptic ulcers.

Daily Norm: No established official norm. The maximum allowable dose in recommendations is 1,000 mg as a complex per day.

Provitamins are compounds that are not active vitamins themselves but can be converted into the active form of a vitamin in the body. They are precursors to vitamins and can ensure their synthesis in the body. Most of those known, in terms of their action, deficiency symptoms, and overdose, are identical to the vitamins they convert into. Therefore, from a practical standpoint, their intake makes sense only when there is some individual intolerance to the base vitamin. The main provitamins known today are provitamin D_3 (7-dehydrocholesterol), provitamin D_2 (ergosterol), provitamin B_3 (tryptophan), provitamin B_5 (panthenol), and provitamin A (beta-carotene), which is worth considering a bit since it has some advantages over vitamin A.

Provitamin A (Beta-Carotene)

Role: A carotenoid that is converted into retinol (vitamin A) in the body. Has potent antioxidant properties, supports eye health, skin, and the immune system.

Symptoms of Possible Deficiency: Dry skin and mucous membranes, night blindness, decreased immunity, growth problems in children.

Symptoms of Overdose: Beta-carotene is considered safe as the body converts it to retinol as needed. Excessive consumption may lead to carotenemia (yellowish skin discoloration), which is not toxic and disappears when intake is reduced.

Synthetic Forms: Synthetic beta-carotene is available as a supplement.

Natural Sources: Carrots, sweet potatoes, pumpkin, spinach, broccoli, apricots, mangoes.

Recommendations for Intake: Take with foods containing fats for better absorption. It's recommended to consume a variety of carotenoid sources from the diet.

<u>Daily Norm:</u> No established official norm for beta-carotene, but consuming 3-7 mg per day is considered to meet the body's necessary needs.

Potentially Beneficial Supplements

If you've read this far, you certainly have intentions to take care of your health, and additional knowledge about interesting beneficial supplements might not be superfluous for you. Unlike essential vitamins and minerals, the intake of all these supplements is not mandatory, but in certain cases, it can be very beneficial. In this section, I will not specify norms or give broad recommendations for most substances because almost all of them do not yet have a sufficient number of representative studies at the moment. However, as experience shows from other people's use, they can be very effective. Therefore, it's sensible to shed some light on this knowledge, and surely there will be someone who can use it to their benefit. You must clearly understand that before starting to take most of these supplements, you should thoroughly research the issue of their action, as some of them have quite specific effects and can have various consequences. That is why, when taking such supplements, you need to monitor your body's reactions more carefully and be more cautious with dosages.

Colostrum is the first milk produced by the mammary glands after birth. It is rich in antibodies, immunoglobulins, and growth factors. Taking colostrum as a supplement can support the immune system, improve gut health, and aid recovery after physical exertion. It is especially popular among athletes and people with increased physical activity.

Invictus Equilibrium

Transfer Factor consists of molecules derived from colostrum, which are believed to influence the immune system. Some studies suggest that they can modulate immune responses and help the body fight infections. Research is still limited, and some studies have conflicts of interest, but they plausibly show the effectiveness of this supplement and the absence of side effects, which generally seems truthful, considering the origin of this supplement.

Trace Minerals are microelements required by the body in small quantities for normal functioning. They include iron, zinc, copper, selenium, gold, silver, and many others. Supplements with trace minerals can help fill deficiencies of microelements, supporting immunity, metabolism, and overall health. It's important to consider that an excess of some microelements can be harmful, but obtaining it in this variant is not easy. For example, my supplement contains 90 different elements at only 4 mg, which is actually not much but can help cover small needs for specific microelements.

Glutathione is a powerful antioxidant synthesized in the body that protects cells from oxidative stress. It plays an important role in liver detoxification and immune system maintenance. Taking glutathione in supplement form can increase antioxidant protection levels.

Cordyceps is a mushroom used in traditional Chinese medicine. It can increase energy and endurance, support lung and kidney function. Some studies indicate its potential ability to improve athletic performance and have immunomodulating properties. Cordyceps may also have antioxidant and anti-inflammatory effects.

Lion's Mane Mushroom is known for its potential neuroprotective properties. It can stimulate the synthesis of nerve growth factor (NGF), supporting the health of the nervous system. Taking supplements with this mushroom can improve cognitive functions, memory, and mood. Some studies also mention its possible benefits in neurodegenerative diseases.

Quercetin is a flavonoid with antioxidant and anti-inflammatory properties. It can support the immune system, reduce allergic reactions, and improve cardiovascular health.

Quercetin is also being studied for its potential antiviral activity.

Resveratrol is an antioxidant found in red wine, grapes, and some berries. It can promote heart health, protect blood vessels, and reduce inflammatory processes. Resveratrol is also being researched for its possible role in slowing down aging processes.

Curcumin is the active component of turmeric, known for its powerful anti-inflammatory and antioxidant properties. It can help with joint diseases, support digestion, and improve brain function. It also exhibits rejuvenating properties, and there is convincing evidence that it can help with depression and chronic pain. Curcumin itself has low bioavailability, so it is often combined with black pepper and/or lipids.

L-Theanine is an amino acid found in green tea. It can promote relaxation, improve concentration, and reduce stress levels without causing drowsiness. The combination of L-theanine with caffeine can enhance cognitive functions. There is an observed effect of reducing anxiety and depression, but data is limited and not 100% scientifically confirmed.

Meldonium is a compound used to improve energy metabolism in cells. It can increase endurance, improve recovery after physical exertion, and support the cardiovascular system. However, meldonium is banned in sports as doping, and its use should be cautious because a list of side effects exists, though they occur rarely. A good option for its use can be in various heart diseases, in the treatment of alcoholism, and to accelerate rehabilitation in the postoperative period.

Ashwagandha is an herb used in Ayurvedic medicine. It can help the body adapt to stress, reduce cortisol levels, improve mood, and support the immune system.

TA-65 is a dietary supplement positioned as a means to support health and slow down aging processes by activating the enzyme telomerase. Telomerase is responsible for maintaining and lengthening telomeres - the end sections of chromosomes that shorten with each cell division. It is believed that telomere shortening is associated with cellular aging and the aging of the body as a whole. This supplement consists of a substance extracted from the root of Astragalus membranaceus. An extract of astragalus root can be purchased separately, and its effect should be similar in essence. The question is only in the concentrations of the elements that provide this effect, and in fact, TA-65 is like a transfer factor made from colostrum - a high concentration of a specific element that scientists today consider key in the root of astragalus. From the studies I've seen, the results are interesting, but data is limited, and there may be a conflict of interest.

Collagen is the main protein of connective tissue, which provides the structure of the skin, bones, cartilage, and ligaments. Collagen makes up about 30% of all proteins in the human body. Taking collagen supplements can improve skin condition, increase its elasticity, and reduce wrinkles. Some studies also indicate possible benefits for joint health, reducing pain, and improving mobility in people with osteoarthritis. Unfortunately, after 25 years, the processes of collagen synthesis in our body begin to slow down, and its overall level starts to decline. Therefore, taking collagen supplements on a permanent basis can potentially bring considerable benefits. There is no set intake norm, and essentially no side effects (the main side effects are related to allergies to the raw materials from which a particular type of collagen is made), because it's essentially an ordinary protein that has been maximally broken down into individual amino acids for optimal absorption. It's also worth adding that collagen is much better absorbed together with vitamin C.

Omega-3 Fatty Acids (EPA and DHA) are important for heart, brain, and eye health. They can reduce inflammation levels, support the cardiovascular system, and improve cognitive functions. Sources of omega-3 are fish oil, flaxseed oil, and chia seeds. This supplement will actually be very beneficial for most people in the modern world, but there is a certain nuance that is better understood. The important thing is not the intake of omega-3 (it can be harmful), but the balance of omega-3 to omega-6. Omega-6 fatty acids are found in large quantities in sunflower, corn, and soybean oils, which are quite abundant in most people's diets today, creating an imbalance that is the root of problems. The normal balance of omega-3 to omega-6 is from 1:1 to 1:4. Statistical data shows that for most people, this balance can reach 1:15 or even 1:20. For example, in my region, sunflower oil is used everywhere, so I personally take omega-3 constantly, although I try to reduce the intake of omega-6.

Intake of Vitamins and Minerals

We need to start by stating that all recommendations and norms for the intake of vitamins and minerals are conditional. Even in different countries, norms can vary significantly. If we take any of the best studies, for example, on the benefits of vitamin D intake, and it proves that taking vitamin D is statistically beneficial, even in such studies, there will always be those who did not receive the expected positive result at all or received a negative one. There will just be few such people, and they will have a very insignificant impact on the overall sample. But they will be there. A norm is not a point you must necessarily reach. A norm is a starting point from which you can push off in search of personal truth. That is why I don't see much sense in writing extensively about the compatibility and incompatibility of simultaneous intake of certain vitamins and minerals. All this information is quite conditional, and it's not difficult to find if needed. There are various tables and articles. My task is to show that there is a problem with the quantity of vitamins and minerals in the modern person's diet. And this problem is actually much bigger than most people think. I'm just planting a seed. How you use the sprouts is your personal business. It's important to understand that current medical norms of anything are not actual norms based on science, but merely indications of trends currently present in the world.

I also believe that our body is very adaptive, and in great need, theoretically, our microbiota can adapt to any compounds, their forms, and quantities (if the intake of such occurs on a permanent basis). The question here is only at what cost to the body these adaptations will occur. Simply knowing certain recommendations can significantly increase efficiency and speed up the process of forming your unique supplement intake formula. Even taking vitamin-mineral complexes, which I consider far from the best option, can be quite beneficial for certain people. It's fair to say that in addition to a sufficiently large number of studies showing their effectiveness close to zero, there is also a sufficient number of studies showing quite high effectiveness from taking vitamin-mineral complexes.

In reality, everything is super individual. Regarding the compatibility of simultaneous intake of vitamins and minerals, everything is very ambiguous and confusing. In my opinion, I did not find completely reliable data. There are studies showing that certain vitamins cannot be taken together because absorption drops significantly. Another does not confirm the same effect. The only thing I've noted is that when taking high dosages of certain vitamins or minerals together, incompatibility effects are more possible than with small dosages. If we look at the issue of compatibility from the point of view of nature, we will find many familiar products for our

Invictus Equilibrium

body in which, according to many doctors, studies, and media personalities, incompatible vitamins and minerals are present together. And I don't think that nature hasn't found a way over millions of years to solve the problem of simultaneous absorption of certain vitamins and minerals. Here, the question is only that certain elements can start reacting with each other even before they reach your stomach, and it makes sense to simply space out their intake over time.

Individual incompatibilities of specific forms of vitamins in specific microbiome environments are certainly possible, but this does not apply to everyone. Therefore, in this matter, I see for myself the only adequate option until there are exact reliable data: try to take all supplements separately. It seems to me that it's better to take a triple dosage once every three days than three elements simultaneously. This is especially true for fat-soluble vitamins and minerals. In my opinion, there is a certain chemical conflict of interest in the simultaneous absorption of fat-soluble vitamins and minerals, especially if we are talking about slightly increased dosages.

In essence, fat-soluble vitamins can be taken together. The question is only whether there will be enough fat in the meal for their absorption. Here I mean that if you are taking large doses of different fat-soluble vitamins, it would be rational to consume them separately in different meals so that they compete less with each other and their absorption increases.

With water-soluble vitamins, I see no problem in simultaneous intake. In general, in my opinion, the actual presence of some deficiency will play an important role. If there is an existing deficiency, your body will definitely make more efforts to cover it, and the "broth" in which you will deliver that vitamin or mineral may play a much smaller role than in the absence of a deficiency when your body has more choices. That is, I think that from a tablet with ten vitamins, the one that will be absorbed best is the vitamin whose deficiency is greatest in the body. I cannot confirm this thought scientifically. There's just a feeling that our body is extraordinarily adaptive, and under different conditions, it can evaluate differently the balance between the energy expended on processing some form of a mineral, for example, and the potential benefits obtained from this mineral. Therefore, in most cases, a bad form will be much better than nothing.

It's also slightly better to take minerals separately because certain forms of them can react with each other and with vitamins, which by their nature are quite active substances. Although studies on the degradation of minerals and mineral complexes indicate that with proper storage (without unnecessary contact with light, air, and moisture), the destruction of minerals almost does not occur, but still, chemistry has not been canceled, and when minerals enter a moist specific environment in the mouth, reactions between them are more possible even before reaching the stomach. Here we can immediately add that the situation with the storage of vitamins is worse than with the storage of minerals. Even with proper storage, vitamins slowly decompose and lose their properties. I have not found anything to indicate that vitamins can become harmful over time. The only possible danger in consuming expired vitamins is the formation of mold or fungi if they were stored in high humidity.

In general, the absorption of vitamins and minerals will strongly depend on the organism into which they enter, but there are common factors for everyone that can greatly reduce their bioavailability. Taking medications very often leads to accelerated loss of vitamins and minerals by the body. Also, genetic deviations can reduce the absorption of a specific vitamin or mineral, which will lead to a constant deficiency and the need for frequent monitoring and intake of increased dosages. Experienced stress can lead to rapid exhaustion of the body. Also, with age, absorption may decline, and increased doses will often be rational. We should not forget that sports also contribute to increased consumption of the body's resources.

Regarding the best time and method of taking vitamins and minerals, nothing specific can be said. In nature, we actually get everything during meals. And it turns out that it's better to add everything to food, but there are small nuances to increase efficiency. With a large amount of fat in the diet, minerals are absorbed slightly worse. This is especially true for magnesium, iron, calcium, and zinc. Minerals, in general, can quite actively react with food components, forming insoluble compounds that will simply be excreted by the body. Therefore, chelated forms are slightly better taken between meals. They are already bound to a certain protein or amino acid, so their additional presence is not necessary. Non-chelated forms are better taken with food because they still need to bind to something for transportation.

I actually believe that in today's world, taking supplements is mandatory. As science shows, it's now easier than ever to get a deficiency, and as practice shows, deficiencies more often bring more harm than excesses. Our body has quite effective mechanisms for eliminating an excess of a specific vitamin or mineral. But if you have a deficiency of something, internal mechanisms to cover it in most cases simply do not exist. From this, we can conclude that with prophylactic doses (30%–80% of the total daily norm) of supplements, it's not easy to harm yourself, but

Invictus Equilibrium

obtaining significant benefits from their intake by simply returning yourself to normal is quite likely.

The main question for me, which is not revealed in most studies: "Does the positive effect of a particular vitamin or mineral occur due to returning to normal or due to the beneficial action of the vitamin or mineral?" And from this follows the question: "Is the use of high doses of a particular vitamin or mineral actually effective?" Since we are all different, we can assume that the norm for all of us is also different, and the effect of large doses of a certain vitamin or mineral on one person can be maximally positive, and on another, maximally negative. In reality, determining these maximally effective doses can only be done experimentally on oneself (but it's worth doing this quite carefully if we're talking about really high dosages). Therefore, the most adequate option at the moment (until some super device is invented that will measure the individual norm for everyone) is to constantly add those vitamins and minerals to your diet that, in your opinion, are simply insufficient in your diet.

It should also be said that the issue of deficiency is somewhat conditional. For example, if under some potent drug your reaction speed increased, you cannot say that you have a deficiency of this drug. An obvious deficiency can be spoken of when there are clear symptoms of a lack of a specific vitamin or mineral. The question is different. When you simply have little energy, slight drowsiness, or irritability, are these features of your character or already existing manifestations of some deficiency (or a combination of several minor deficiencies)? In reality, there is no clear symptom that can be said to definitively indicate some deficiency. We are all different, and we can all have different symptoms of this or that. But the presence of some symptom should prompt us to certain reflections and possibly conduct additional research of our body, but now with a probably more accurate identification of the problem.

My personal approach to taking vitamins and minerals is somewhat chaotic, but in essence, that's how it happens in nature anyway. In fact, I have most of all the necessary vitamins and minerals for the body (currently 16 different supplements). Of these supplements, I am currently systematically taking only vitamins A and E because their levels in my blood are close to deficient, and I have exact test results. Everything else I just periodically add to my diet. Simply in each meal, I take 2–3 compatible supplements in prophylactic dosages, constantly changing them. And what is better taken without food, I usually take before workouts, which allows for slightly increased absorption because physical activity actively increases blood circulation and, as a result, the speed of metabolism.

Invictus Equilibrium

In conclusion, I want to say that I do not believe that vitamins and minerals have some miraculous effect and can cure any diseases. For me personally, this is a way to return my body to normal working mode. Here, the question arises about the real capabilities of our body. Most likely, a large amount of energy, high efficiency, normal sleep, absence of diseases, and the like are the normal functioning of our body, which most of us have already forgotten and which does not strongly coincide with the realities of the modern world.

Tests and Analyses

Technology today is advancing so rapidly that it leads to its quick dissemination and penetration into the lives of the masses. And this is definitely worth taking advantage of. Modern methods of analyzing various parts of our body allow us to obtain a huge amount of quite accurate data, which can facilitate the search for weak spots in your body. And all this is becoming more accessible every day.

For example, by conducting a screening of the elemental composition of hair, you can draw many conclusions about deficiencies or excesses of certain elements in your body. Hair is not a storage of minerals, but with its analysis, conclusions can be made about the presence of minerals in the body at the time of growth.

It should also be understood that the results of analyses can have deviations, and this is normal (regardless of the accuracy declared by the laboratory). In different laboratories, the same hair will, in most cases, have slightly different results. This is influenced by an extremely large number of random factors during calculation. Particularly large inaccuracies can occur when taking tests for various hormones. Their levels in our body change constantly. If you were a bit nervous before the test, your entire hormonal

Invictus Equilibrium

background changed. Therefore, it's very important to approach testing quite seriously. Do it under the same conditions to increase accuracy. But bad data in most cases will be much better than their absence and will serve as a good foundation for researching your body.

It's impossible to say that some analyses are more important than others; everything is situational. But for periodic preventive monitoring of your overall health level, a general blood test, immunogram, levels of fat-soluble vitamins D, A, and E, urine analysis, coprogram, and proteinogram are well suited. It is recommended to check your body at least once a year. But in fact, if absolutely nothing bothers you and your age is quite young, examinations can be conducted at longer intervals. The question is how well you understand your body's signals. Previously, medicine didn't exist at all. But it's fair to say that people lived a bit less.

Taking tests for water-soluble vitamins doesn't make much sense because they do not accumulate and can be completely excreted from the blood in 1–3 days. In fact, the result will heavily depend on what you ate yesterday.

In analyses, much depends not so much on the numbers they will have but on the correct interpretation. And here you either need to delve a bit into this topic yourself or consult a qualified doctor. But if you at least figure out hormones and vitamins, you can solve a large number of problems and subsequently independently control these values.

Chapter 14
Stress

"Save yourself, and thousands will be saved around you."

Sergey Radonezhsky

The modern world is filled with various stimuli that affect our psyche. The age at which different psychological illnesses manifest is rapidly decreasing. For example, there are about 4 times more people aged 18–25 diagnosed with depression compared to those over 50[1]. If you take a close look at the things that surround us today, you'll find that most of them are completely unnatural for us. By understanding, even a little, how the most ordinary things around us affect our mental health, you can make your life a bit brighter.

Rest

Let's start with the fact that rest is at least the absence of work. In today's world, there are many people who work a lot. Research shows that after 4 hours of concentrated work, productivity starts to decline significantly. Even if you work with breaks, after 50 hours of work per week (if you maintain this schedule continuously), real productivity can even become negative. Those who constantly work more than 64 hours per week accomplish less than those who work 56 hours. That is, everything beyond 50 hours of work per week for most people will have a negative effect[2]. Therefore, one of the best ways to combat stress is to work less.

As animals, nature is extremely important to us. This is actually a fundamental thing necessary for our normal existence. No matter how you look at it, we are creatures of nature. Studies show that even briefly listening to birdsong, the sound of the sea, or just gazing at a green tree improves our productivity. Even a small contact with nature seems to reboot our brain[3,4].

Our brain is structured in such a way that it cannot relax in an urban environment. Even a walk around the city does not lead to psychological relaxation. The constant, varied noise of the city, the sharp lines of buildings, the endless flow of other people - none of this allows our nervous system to relax and keeps it constantly tense. Perhaps this is because our brain evolved under completely opposite conditions (lots of light, vast open landscapes, a very different and much lower noise load, small communities). Even short stays in areas with plenty of greenery calm our psyche and improve cognitive abilities. Children who spend little time in green spaces show an increased rate of psychological disorders (children almost never suffer from psychological illnesses, which is generally atypical for them). Patients in hospitals whose windows overlook green plantations recover faster than those whose windows face urban development[5]. In areas where forests have disappeared due to certain cataclysms, there's an observed increase in various diseases. Even statistically, the favorite colors of most people on the planet are blue and green (sea and grass?). Asphalt, iron, brick, glass, etc. - all of these are very unnatural for our psyche. Spend more time in nature and feel yourself as part of it. More specifically, positive changes in the body are observed after just two hours per week spent in nature[6].

A simple walk in the forest very beneficially affects our immunity. Forest air has a high concentration of phytoncides, which activate our immune system, reduce cortisol levels, and help normalize blood pressure. The greatest production of phytoncides occurs in coniferous forests during the warm season. And what would happen if you started running in coniferous forests?

They also say that meditation helps unload the mind and reboot the brain. But I personally do not practice it. I believe you need to be quite cautious with it. Meditation is, to some extent, immersion into oneself, and there are plenty of documented cases where people lost their minds after beginning regular meditation practices. One cannot argue that there are also many people who benefit from it. Therefore, if you plan to practice it, I advise you to approach its study very seriously and make conclusions for yourself after thorough research.

Social Networks

Social networks today are one of the most massive drugs on the planet (if not the most massive). And this is no joke. They really cause a stable addiction, confirmed by numerous studies. If you compare the brain reactions of a heroin addict and a person who spends a lot of time on social networks, they are almost identical[7].

I've already written that social networks break our reward system, but unfortunately, that's not all the negative effects. They also strongly influence our psyche and can lead to a host of nervous disorders.

We are used to living in a hierarchical society, and our brain is constantly trying to understand where we stand in this hierarchical society and where everyone else stands. If we consider a primitive tribe, in most cases, among 100 people,

Invictus Equilibrium

there were 2–3 of higher rank (the chief and assistants), 2–3 of lower rank (the weakest), and the main mass who were not very different from each other. This means that in such a social group, no great psychological pressure is created on the absolute majority because almost everyone is conditionally equal. A similar principle was and is found in most other social structures (work, school, country, etc.). Today, however, those who spend time on social networks subconsciously compare themselves with others and, in most cases, see lives better than their own. As a result, this can cause addiction, depression, panic attacks, increased anxiety, insomnia, etc. For the not yet fully formed mind of a child, this has an even stronger impact than on adults.

In summary, it's better to give up social networks or at least minimize their use if they are not related to your work. It's better to start communicating more with live people. This actually significantly reduces stress. We are all extremely social organisms and need live communication. For example, simple hugs trigger the release of oxytocin in our brains, which calms us and makes us happier. But if you are firmly convinced that you are not addicted to social networks, just delete them all from your phone for one week, and in most cases, you'll be convinced otherwise. And regarding the beautiful life of everyone on social networks except you—this is actually an illusion. Everyone posts only their best photos, which do not reflect the realities of life. These are all constructed images. In reality, such ideal people simply do not exist. It's all untrue! Even princesses use the toilet.

Sports and Stress

Regular physical activity is very important for the normal functioning of our body, and I have already written a lot about it. But there are small nuances regarding its effect on stress levels, which should be clarified.

In general, physical activity is stress for our body, but on the other hand, it helps release stress and teaches our body to adapt to it. A lot depends on the initial level of stress and the choice of sport you engage in. It's very important, for reducing stress, to choose an activity in which you will focus your thoughts on your body and not be able to think about the source of stress (a bad boss, a broken car, etc.). For example, I love playing volleyball, and during the game, I simply cannot think of anything other than the ball. I've often asked myself what I think about during the game, and the answer has always been the same: I think about the game and nothing else that happens around me.

It's also proven that "fidgeting" or "tinkering", "grinding" with something helps reduce stress[8,9]. It's not fully understood how this works, but everyone has noticed that in

Invictus Equilibrium

stressful situations, you want to rub your hands, tap your fingers on something, bite your nails, tap or shake your legs, etc. Maybe this is related to the nervous system's desire to shift attention from some nerve impulses to others, thus getting through the present stress. Essentially, sports also fit well into the category of "fidgeting" stress away. This category can also include biting objects, clicking, chewing, and similar behaviors.

Another way to influence stress levels can be various breathing practices. There are a huge number of them, and they can have different effects (calming, exciting, increasing concentration, etc.). There are even studies showing that breathing by the Wim Hof method can increase immunity. His practices are actually quite interesting. He has, in laboratory conditions, demonstrated that he can control hormonal reactions in his body and claims he can teach this to anyone (and in essence, he does), and it even seems plausible.

But personally, I see certain nuances in such practices. I also believe that one can learn, within certain limits, to control the body's internal reactions and maybe Wim Hof's techniques are one way to do this. However, I also believe that nothing in this world is free. If you somehow managed at a certain moment to mobilize more energy than your body initially allowed, it most likely happened at the expense of some internal energy reserves. You simply took from one place and put it into another, creating the illusion of increased energy, although you didn't add anything from outside. Therefore, from this point of view, I believe that such practices have the right to exist. Understanding and being able to at least slightly consciously control your internal energy can give you many potential advantages and self-confidence. But you must use this knowledge and skill quite carefully and with full awareness of why you are doing it. Personally, I practiced some breathing exercises from yoga for a while (yoga also helps reduce stress levels) and I even managed to slightly control my heartbeat.

The Conditional Nature of the World

All our feelings and emotions are conditional. Everything around you is conditional. Love, happiness, joy - all these are conditional values that cannot be measured. This applies not only to psychological components but also to physical ones. The world a color-blind person sees is definitely different from what you see. But if a color-blind person were never told that everyone else sees the world differently, he wouldn't suspect that his world isn't "normal." A person blind from birth considers his world "normal" until someone explains that his world is incomplete. In childhood, a stick, a puddle, and a bug were enough to make us happy, but in adulthood, it doesn't always work that way. This only proves that the brightness of the world around you depends much more on your perception than on the actual state of things.

There is a lot of research proving that emotions from failures are stronger than emotions from successes. That is, you will experience much more anxiety when you lose $1,000,000 than when you win $1,000,000.[10] Logically, it seems that the emotional component should be the same, but science says we more strongly experience negative emotions than positive ones. This is our evolutionary adaptation, so we better remember life-threatening situations. Marketing skillfully uses this. Today's world is full of negativity and countless things that constantly destabilize your psyche and make you think that you are somehow incomplete and that someone else knows better how you should live your life and what you should strive for. Today's pace of life forces most people to be under constant stress, leading to a host of negative health consequences and making people unhappy. In reality, NOBODY knows what is right. The norm does not exist! It was invented. In the past, it was normal to burn a woman in the city square and everyone applauded. Now the norms are slightly different. But the question is whether the "normal" life imposed on you as a norm is actually your desire. I'm not suggesting to go back to burning women in the city square. I'm just saying maybe you should stop worrying about what you cannot influence. "Do what you must, and let what will be, be!" as the ancient Roman Emperor Marcus Aurelius said.

The conditionality of our life is accidental. None of us chose where or when to be born. No one chose their gender, the shape of their nose, etc. If you think about it, our whole life is an endless sequence of coincidences, and our influence on this chain of events is actually minimal. That's why there's no point in worrying about where you've ended up. It has already happened. Fill your life with positive emotions. Discard everything that is imposed on you. Think about what you really want from this life and why it was given to you. Try to find your true goal and reach it. But if you achieve something else, maybe you just misunderstood your goal. We all ended up here by chance and at the same time not by chance. Each of us in this world can do anything that does not violate the boundaries of others. Do what you want, but never forget to remain human.

Afterword

Today, 80% of the planet's population lives better than 99% of all the kings and queens who ever existed. This is not obvious, but most of us have already become so accustomed to showers, toilets, three meals a day, movie theaters, cars, airplanes, delivery services, and an immense variety of foods that we consider it normal. Yet just about 100 years ago, things were completely different. New knowledge and technologies have brought a great deal of benefit to our large Homo Sapiens family, but on the other hand, it is now extremely easy to get confused and lose yourself in this infinity of information and comfort. No one knows where we are all heading. And no one knows which road is the right one.

That is why I would like to wish everyone who reads this book to find their own path. Everyone's is unique. Each person must learn their own lessons from it. And to make your path easier, I suggest you create your own checklist of things you'd like to change. Don't put it off. Start right now. Just take a blank piece of paper and develop your own specific plan, which you will break down into a large number of small innovations. And gradually introduce all of this into your life.

Before you know it, by taking very small steps, you will be able to achieve the highest goals.

Because, as it seems to me, with a clear mind and a healthy body, it will be a bit easier to find yourself in this world. I hope that my work will help you find your life's path a little faster. Good luck!

Sources

I would very much have liked to list all the information sources I used when writing this book, but unfortunately, some of the scientific data I wrote down came straight from my head. This does not mean that there are no actual studies and that I made everything up. It's just that I read a certain number of scientific works long before I planned to write this book and could not find all the original sources again. However, I am leaving references for most of the data.

If any of you genuinely wish to check the relevance of the information on the topics discussed in this book and do not know where to look for scientific articles, great resources for searching scientific papers include: scholar.google.com, pubmed.ncbi.nlm.nih.gov, ncbi.nlm.nih.gov, sci-hub.se. I should also mention that some basic information was taken from the resource wikipedia.org.

I am certain that there are enough new studies on the topics I covered, and it's possible that new data in some areas may even refute what I have written. But the only one who never makes mistakes is the one who does nothing at all.

Chapter 2. Evolution Is Killing You

1. https://worldostats.com/life-expectancy-by-country-2024/

2. https://en.wikipedia.org/wiki/Pure%2C_White_and_Deadly

3. Thomas G. Travison et al., 2007 "A Population-Level Decline in Serum Testosterone Levels in American Men".

4. Ying Chen et al., 2022 "National Data on Age Gradients in Well-being Among US Adults".

Chapter 3. Basics

1. Eleanor Klibaner-Schiff et al., 2024 "Environmental exposures influence multigenerational epigenetic transmission".

2. https://en.wikipedia.org/wiki/%C3%96verkalix_study (Överkalix study)

3. Valorie N Salimpoor et al., 2011 "Anatomically distinct dopamine release during anticipation and experience of peak emotion to music".

4. Karen M Grewen et al., 2003 "Warm partner contact is related to lower cardiovascular reactivity".

5. Sheldon Cohen et al., 2014 "Does Hugging Provide Stress-Buffering Social Support? A Study of Susceptibility to Upper Respiratory Infection and Illness".

6. Tristen K Inagaki et al., 2012 "Neural correlates of giving support to a loved one".

Invictus Equilibrium

7. https://en.wikipedia.org/wiki/Hygiene_hypothesis

Chapter 4. The Brain

1. Martin Shepperd et al., 2018 "An Experimental Evaluation of a De-biasing Intervention for Professional Software Developers".

2. Phillippa Lally et al., 2009 "How are habits formed: Modelling habit formation in the real world".

3. Keara E. Valentine et al., 2019 "The Efficacy of Hypnosis as a Treatment for Anxiety: A Meta-Analysis".

4. Curt P. Richter, 1957 "On the Phenomenon of Sudden Death in Animals and Man".

5. Victoria J. Rideout et al., 2010 "Generation M^2: Media in the Lives of 8- to 18-Year-Olds".

6. Adrian F. Ward et al., 2017 "Brain Drain: The Mere Presence of One's Own Smartphone Reduces Available Cognitive Capacity".

7. Kyung Hee Kim, 2011 "The Creativity Crisis: The Decrease in Creative Thinking Scores on the Torrance Tests of Creative Thinking".

8. Bernt Bratsberg et al., 2018 "Flynn effect and its reversal are both environmentally caused".

9. Zubair Ahmed Ratan et al., 2021 "Smartphone Addiction and Associated Health Outcomes in Adult Populations: A Systematic Review".

10. Yehuda Wacks et al., 2021 "Excessive Smartphone Use Is Associated With Health Problems in Adolescents and Young Adults".

11. Cunjia Liu, 2023 "The unique role of smartphone addiction and related factors among university students: a model based on cross-sectional and cross-lagged network analyses".

Chapter 5. Sleep

1. Tian-Shu Zheng et al., 2024 "Sleep deprivation stimulates adaptive thermogenesis by activating AMPK pathway in mice".

2. Ben Korin et al., 2019 "Short-term sleep deprivation in mice induces B cell migration to the brain compartment ".

3. https://en.wikipedia.org/wiki/Sleep_deprivation

4. Andrew D. Nguyen et al., 2024 "A perfect storm: sleep loss causes systemic inflammation and death".

5. Jean-Philippe Chaput et al., 2020 "Sleep Duration and Health in Adults: An Overview of Systematic Reviews".

6. Siaw Cheok Liew et al., 2020 "Sleep deprivation and its association with diseases- a review".

7. Sergio Garbarino et al., 2021 "Role of sleep deprivation in immune-related disease risk and outcomes".

8. Daoyun Ji et al., 2007 "Coordinated memory replay in the visual cortex and hippocampus during sleep".

9. Suzanne Dawson et al., 2024 "Weighted Blankets as a Sleep Intervention: A Scoping Review".

10. Bodil Ekholm et al., 2020 "A randomized controlled study of weighted chain blankets for insomnia in psychiatric disorders".

Chapter 8. Water

1. Karine Keyzy dos Santos Lemes Lechuga et al., 2023 "Music and Tactile Stimuli during Daily Milking Affect the Welfare and Productivity of Dairy Cows".

Chapter 9. Air

1. Dieter Lüthi et al., 2008 "High-resolution carbon dioxide concentration record 650,000–800,000 years before present".

2. Joseph G. Allen et al., 2015 "Associations of Cognitive Function Scores with Carbon Dioxide, Ventilation, and Volatile Organic Compound Exposures in Office Workers: A Controlled Exposure Study of Green and Conventional Office Environments".

3. https://www.epa.gov/iaq-schools/research-references-related-indoor-air-quality-schools

4. Jose Guillermo Cedeño Laurent et al., 2021 "Associations between acute exposures to PM2.5 and carbon dioxide indoors and cognitive function in office workers: a multicountry longitudinal prospective observational study".

5. Nuno Canha et al., 2021 "How Is Indoor Air Quality during Sleep? A Review of Field Studies".

6. Jing Wang et al., 2024 "Associations between indoor fine particulate matter (PM2.5) and sleep-disordered breathing in an urban sample of school-aged children".

Chapter 10. Body

1. Dana R. Carney et al., 2010 "Power Posing: Brief Nonverbal Displays Affect Neuroendocrine Levels and Risk Tolerance".

2. Marie P. Cross et al., 2021 "How and why could smiling influence physical health? A conceptual review".

3. David George Behm et al., 2023 "Acute Effects of Various Stretching Techniques on Range of Motion: A Systematic Review with Meta-Analysis".

4. Zheng Ke et al., 2011 "The Effects of Voluntary, Involuntary, and Forced Exercises on Brain-Derived Neurotrophic Factor and Motor Function Recovery: A Rat Brain Ischemia Model".

5. Alfonso J. Alfini et al., 2016 "Hippocampal and Cerebral Blood Flow after Exercise Cessation in Master Athletes".

6. P Srámek et al., 2000 "Human physiological responses to immersion into water of different temperatures".

7. Mark J W Hanssen et al., 2015 "Short-term cold acclimation improves insulin sensitivity in patients with type 2 diabetes mellitus".

8. Mark Russell et al., 2017 "The Effects of a Single Whole-Body Cryotherapy Exposure on Physiological, Performance,

and Perceptual Responses of Professional Academy Soccer Players After Repeated Sprint Exercise".

9. Gráinne M. Fitzsimons et al., 2008 "Automatic Effects of Brand Exposure on Motivated Behavior: How Apple Makes You "Think Different"".

10. Paul C Bernhardt et al., 1998 "Testosterone changes during vicarious experiences of winning and losing among fans at sporting events".

11. Chris Baumann et al., 2016 "School discipline, school uniforms and academic performance".

12. Elisabetta Gentile et al., 2009 "Dressed for Success: Do School Uniforms Improve Student Behavior, Attendance, and Achievement?".

13. Warren G. Sanger et al., 1989 "Fit of underwear and male spermatogenesis: A pilot investigation".

14. Donald L. Hilton Jr., 2013 "Pornography addiction – a supranormal stimulus considered in the context of neuroplasticity".

Chapter 11. Nutrition

1. Ta-Chiang Liu et al., 2021 "Western diet induces Paneth cell defects through microbiome alterations and farnesoid X receptor and type I interferon activation".

2. Danziger S et al., 2011 "Extraneous factors in judicial decisions.".

3. https://www.who.int/news-room/fact-sheets/detail/salt-reduction

4. Phillip A Engen et al., 2015 "The Gastrointestinal Microbiome. Alcohol Effects on the Composition of Intestinal Microbiota".

5. L. Segovia-Rodríguez et al., 2022 "Gut microbiota and voluntary alcohol consumption".

6. Javier I. Borráz-León et al., 2022 "Are Toxoplasma-infected subjects more attractive, symmetrical, or healthier than non-infected ones? Evidence from subjective and objective".

7. Joe Alcock et al., 2014 "Is eating behavior manipulated by the gastrointestinal microbiota? Evolutionary pressures and potential mechanisms".

8. Katherine Dinan et al., 2022 "Antibiotics and mental health: The good, the bad and the ugly".

9. ME Glover et al., 2021 "Examining the role of microbiota in emotional behavior: antibiotic treatment exacerbates anxiety in high anxiety-prone male rats.".

Invictus Equilibrium

10. John F. Cryan et al., 2019 "The Microbiota-Gut-Brain Axis".

11. John R. Tagg et al., 2023 "Beneficial modulation of human health in the oral cavity and beyond using bacteriocin-like inhibitory substance-producing streptococcal probiotics".

12. David A Wiss et al., 2018 "Sugar Addiction: From Evolution to Revolution".

13. Magalie Lenoir et al., 2007 "Intense Sweetness Surpasses Cocaine Reward".

14. James Ousey et al., 2023 "Gut microbiota suppress feeding induced by palatable foods".

15. Nallely Bueno-Hernández et al., 2020 "Chronic sucralose consumption induces elevation of serum insulin in young healthy adults: a randomized, double blind, controlled trial".

16. Dominika Głąbska et al., 2020 "Fruit and Vegetable Intake and Mental Health in Adults: A Systematic Review".

17. Hajara Aslam et al., 2024 "Fiber intake and fiber intervention in depression and anxiety: a systematic review and meta-analysis of observational studies and randomized controlled trials".

18. Sydney E. Martin et al., 2023 "The Role of Diet on the Gut Microbiome, Mood and Happiness".

19. William E Kraus et al., 2020 "Two Years of Calorie Restriction and Cardiometabolic Risk Factors".

20. Noni L. Bodkin et al., 2003 "Mortality and Morbidity in Laboratory-maintained Rhesus Monkeys and Effects of Long-term Dietary Restriction".

21. María Morales-Suarez-Varela et al., 2021 "Intermittent Fasting and the Possible Benefits in Obesity, Diabetes, and Multiple Sclerosis: A Systematic Review of Randomized Clinical Trials".

22. Michael Albosta et al., 2021 "Intermittent fasting: is there a role in the treatment of diabetes? A review of the literature and guide for primary care physicians".

23. https://en.wikipedia.org/wiki/Anti-aging_movement

24. Ou Fu et al., 2019 "Hypothalamic neuronal circuits regulating hunger-induced taste modification".

25. Ruijuan Liu et al., 2024 "Characterizing the photodegradation-induced release of volatile organic compounds from bottled water containers".

26. Vishal Afreen et al., 2023 "Adverse health effects and mechanisms of microplastics on female reproductive system: a descriptive review".

27. Chen Zhang et al., 2024 "Association of mixed exposure to microplastics with sperm dysfunction: a multi-site study in China".

28. Naveen Kumar et al., 2024 "Microplastics – A Growing Concern as Carcinogens in Cancer Etiology: Emphasis on Biochemical and Molecular Mechanisms".

29. https://en.wikipedia.org/wiki/Endocrine_disruptor

30. Chun Z. Yang et al., 2011 "Most Plastic Products Release Estrogenic Chemicals: A Potential Health Problem that Can Be Solved".

31. John D Meeker et al., 2014 "Urinary phthalate metabolites are associated with decreased serum testosterone in men, women, and children from NHANES 2011-2012".

32. Stephen S. Holden et al., 2015 "Whether Smaller Plates Reduce Consumption Depends on Who's Serving and Who's Looking: A Meta-Analysis".

33. Maria Carlota Dao et al., 2014 "Akkermansia muciniphila and improved metabolic health during a dietary intervention in obesity: relationship with gut microbiome richness and ecology".

34. Yanqing Zhao et al., 2024 "Akkermansia muciniphila: A promising probiotic against inflammation and metabolic disorders".

35. Leila Khalili et al., 2024 "The Role of Akkermansia muciniphila on Improving Gut and Metabolic Health Modulation: A Meta-Analysis of Preclinical Mouse Model Studies".

Chapter 12. Stimulants

1. Johannes Knabbe et al., 2022 "Single-dose ethanol intoxication causes acute and lasting neuronal changes in the brain".

2. Anya Topiwala et al., 2021 "No safe level of alcohol consumption for brain health: observational cohort study of 25,378 UK Biobank participants".

3. Remi Daviet et al., 2022 "Associations between alcohol consumption and gray and white matter volumes in the UK Biobank".

4. Daniel Frings et al., 2020 "Comparison of Allen Carr's Easyway programme with a specialist behavioural and pharmacological smoking cessation support service: a randomized controlled trial"

Chapter 13. Vitamins and Minerals

1. Donald R. Davis, 2009 "Declining Fruit and Vegetable Nutrient Composition: What Is the Evidence?".

2. Raju Lal Bhardwaj et al., 2024 "An Alarming Decline in the Nutritional Quality of Foods: The Biggest Challenge for Future Generations' Health".

3. Food and Agriculture Organization of the United Nations, 1972, FAO Soils Bulletin No. 17, "Trace elements in soils and agriculture."

4. Z. X. Tan et al., 2008 "Global Soil Nutrient Depletion and Yield Reduction".

5. Sangeeta Yadav et al., 2023 "Vitamins and Minerals: A Review on Processing Losses and Strategies to Control It".

6. Emily K. Tarleton et al., 2017 "Role of magnesium supplementation in the treatment of depression: A randomized clinical trial".

7. Mahdi Moabedi et al., 2023 "Magnesium supplementation beneficially affects depression in adults with depressive

disorder: a systematic review and meta-analysis of randomized clinical trials".

8. Danny Phelan et al., 2018 "Magnesium and mood disorders: systematic review and meta-analysis".

https://en.wikipedia.org/wiki/Vitamin

https://en.wikipedia.org/wiki/Mineral_(nutrient)

Chapter 14. Stress

1. https://www.nimh.nih.gov/health/statistics/major-depression

2. John Pencavel, 2014 "The Productivity of Working Hours".

3. Acoustical Society of America (ASA), 2015 "Natural sounds improve mood and productivity".

4. Dianne A. Vella-Brodrick et al., 2022 "Effects of Nature (Greenspace) on Cognitive Functioning in School Children and Adolescents: a Systematic Review".

5. R S Ulrich, 1984 "View through a window may influence recovery from surgery".

6. Mathew P. White et al., 2019 "Spending at least 120 minutes a week in nature is associated with good health and wellbeing".

7. Eszter Áfra et al., 2024 "Altered functional brain networks in problematic smartphone and social media use: resting-state fMRI study".

8. Kadriye Sayin Kasar et al., 2020 "The effect of a stress ball on stress, vital signs and patient comfort in hemodialysis patients: A randomized controlled trial".

9. Elif Gezginci et al., 2018 "Comparison of Two Different Distraction Methods Affecting the Level of Pain and Anxiety during Extracorporeal Shock Wave Lithotripsy: A Randomized Controlled Trial".

10. Alexander L. Brown et al., 2024 "Meta-analysis of Empirical Estimates of Loss Aversion".

Invictus Equilibrium

If anyone has any suggestions, objections, or proposals, you can write to me at dmytrokovalchyk@gmail.com. I do not promise quick responses, but I will periodically check in there.

I've also created an Instagram account, it's currently inactive, but if many of you join, I'll definitely start posting something interesting and useful there: @invictus_diko

If you enjoyed this book, I would be incredibly grateful if you could leave your honest review on Amazon.

If there are those who want to thank me financially, you can do so with cryptocurrency:

BTC (Main)

bc1qfhh6hyz9e3njm3s5sfnyjl8h6243pvyramqxea

Dmytro Kovalchuk

ETH (ERC20)

0x0cb031289cBFa7fAa9a3fb4D215b3fD5A761A160

DOGE (Main)

DLxfbXctQxAcN4Zu5bLToLQdpRd7tjD7ek

Made in the USA
Columbia, SC
04 February 2025